IN THE PRESENCE OF CHENG MAN-CH'ING

My Life And Lessons With The Master Of Five Excellences

WILLIAM C. PHILLIPS

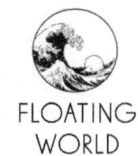

FLOATING WORLD

Copyright © 2019 by William C. Phillips

All rights reserved. No part of this book may be used or reproduced in any manner whatsoever without written permission except in the case of brief quotations embodied in a critical article or review.

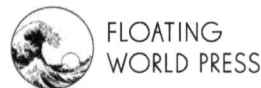

For more information:
contact@floatingworldpress.com
http://www.floatingworldpress.com

Author Information:
William C. Phillips
Patience T'ai Chi Association
PO Box 630001
Bronx NY 10463
Email: sifu@patiencetaichi.com

ISBN 978-0-6482831-2-6

First Edition: December 2019

10 9 8 7 6 5 4 3 2 1

CONTENTS

Preface i

Chapter 1: The Preamble: or What Went Before 1
Chapter 2: Ju Jitsu, Judo and Karate, and How I Learned About T'ai Chi 5
Chapter 3: Stanley Israel at Midwood Dojo 27
Chapter 4: I Begin to Study with Professor Cheng 37
Chapter 5: Permissions and Media 47
Chapter 6: More Stories from the Association 57
Chapter 7: Shr Jung 71
Chapter 8: More Stories from the Shr Jung 95
Chapter 9: Some Reflections on the Senior Students 117
Chapter 10: Fellow Students 127
Chapter 11: The Professor's Wisdom, Teachings and Habits 133
Chapter 12: What I Figured Out for Myself 161
Chapter 13: Self–Defense 183
Chapter 14: Conclusion 201

Final Thank Yous 203
Glossary & Terminology 221
Appendix 1 224
Author's Biography 225

PREFACE

I want to thank everyone who helped me to become who I am today, and by that I mean teachers and students in T'ai Chi and martial arts, as well as my personal friends. I thank the teachers because they taught me something. I thank the students because I taught them something, and in doing so, continued my learning process on the journey of becoming. I thank my friends because they generously shared their ideas, and themselves, with me.

I am indeed a lucky person to have had some of the best teachers, students, and friends, often with people in more than one role at a time.

I was taught how to recognize the multiple roles that a person can have in your life by Dan Millman, author of the book, *Way of the Peaceful Warrior*, who I taught a bit of T'ai Chi to, and who taught me a little about a lot of different things. In this process we became good acquaintances.

To start, I would like to thank Professor Cheng Man-Ch'ing, without whom there would be nothing much to write. He was a great teacher, a great humanitarian, and a wise man. He was very concerned that we learn the T'ai Chi for our health, but also that we learn to be good people. He wanted us to learn how to improve ourselves as we went along. I was in constant awe of him and it was a privilege to have known him. His T'ai Chi skills were so very high, and his dedication to us, his students, was great. He was a master of the traditional Chinese Five Excellences: painting, poetry, calligraphy, medicine and T'ai Chi Ch'uan, as well as of philosophy, and the art of being a good human being.

I thank Katie and Ellen Cheng, (Professor's daughters) who have always been friendly and supportive. They encouraged me in my efforts to remember things from the Association and from the Shr Jung. They also have many wonderful memories of their father (I hope they will write a book of their own some time.) I thank Patrick and Wayne Cheng (Professor's sons) who befriended me in Professor Cheng's school and who I did a demonstration with at the City University of New York Graduate Center. (See pictures). And **I thank Marina Cheng**, (Professor's daughter whose life ended way too soon, and who was teaching me Five Element theory in exchange for some help with her English.)

I thank the late Zhang Lu–Ping who was a friend as well as a teacher from 1988 to 1998. Master Zhang taught me some Yang Long Form and sharpened up my push hands skills as I was still somewhat stiff when I had been studying with Professor Cheng and there was a lot I just could not understand in those days. Professor's senior student Mort Raphael had also tried to teach me some of these things, but I was not ready. Master Zhang found me when I was ready and he gave generously of himself and of his knowledge. Lu–Ping said that "Professor Cheng taught you to be soft, and now I can teach you to be essentially hard. Professor Cheng could not have taught you to be hard, because you would have misinterpreted hard and become tense." Truer words were never spoken. He also told me, "Hurry up and write your book, and I will write a forward for it." But I was young and thought he would be around forever, and so I did not pay attention to this.

I mention here **his son, Huan Zhang**, who has been a friend to me since we met, and who is my T'ai Chi contact person in Massachusetts. Huan is a practitioner of T'ai Chi and a scholar, who has written a book and many articles on T'ai Chi. Huan is a teacher at the University of Massachusetts as of this writing, as well as a T'ai Chi teacher in private practice.

Now I want to come back to the senior students of Professor Cheng, who were also my teachers, and separately thank them:

Mort Raphael, to whom Professor Cheng assigned the impossible task of being my mentor, and of relaxing me so that I could penetrate to the essence of Professor's T'ai Chi and push hands. He worked with me long and hard and I must have been a very difficult assignment. I thank Mort for his friendship, and his deep and ever replenishing well of patience with my tension, and my errors.

Ling Raphael, Mort's wife, to whom I could always turn if I wanted face time and translation with Professor Cheng when Tam Gibbs and Ed Young were getting tired of my incessant questions. I was full of questions. Professor Cheng did not seem to mind, though Tam and Ed sometimes did, telling me that they were concerned for Professor, and wanted to shield him from those of us with too many questions, like me. So Ling would take me to the Professor and translate for me whenever I got too much on Tam or Ed's nerves and they sent me away.

The late **Stan Israel**, who taught me judo and ju jitsu, and showed me Professor's 37 form, starting in February of 1967. He started me on push hands in 1968, and told me about the Professor. Because of Stan, I started my quest for T'ai Chi. Also because of Stan, I decorated the walls of his school with my body as I was pushed into them for hours at a time, late on Saturday afternoons. But more on that later...

The late **Lou Kliensmith** played push hands with me and showed me what push hands could be if it is done softly. We laughed together as I took big hops and little hops, and sometimes flew, crashing into the walls at the Shr Jung. I am now first learning how he did it. The concept is that you can use a small off balance, correctly timed, to push. If done correctly, it can be a thing of joy.

Maggie Newman was there from the start. I did not know her very well until she taught an advanced class and had us students participate as teachers, showing our classmates what T'ai Chi meant to us, and allowing us to strut our stuff. I demonstrated the rooting, or foothold technique. Maggie's advanced class was a successful experiment in democratic T'ai Chi. She is a wonderful, kindly woman and her T'ai Chi has a crystal peace to it that only those energy (ch'i) sensitive souls who experience her doing a round can appreciate.

The late **Tam Gibbs**, Professor's disciple, who traveled with Professor, and was one of those who translated for him at lectures, and talks. He also was (along with Ed) a translator when anyone (I, for example) asked questions. He played sword dueling with me, showing me anew just how stiff I was.

Ed Young, was the other main translator for the Professor. He let me drive him to, and assist at, the Yale T'ai Chi club where I learned some important lessons about how to, and how not to, teach T'ai Chi. Ed Young is also an accomplished artist, and won a Caldecott award.

Both Tam and Ed translated for me when I had questions at the school and also when I picked Professor up on Riverside Drive to transport them to the Association. I am very grateful for that opportunity.

Herman Kauz, who was acting as a de-facto senior student in New York. Herman was kind to me, and stood up for all the senior students and kept the school under its teachers when some students wanted to rebel and lead us astray at the Shr Jung. In Professor's absence, Herman told them that they were there to learn from their betters, and that they were not there to lead their juniors astray.

I've included more thank-you messages at the back of the book along with a glossary of terms for any Asian martial arts terms the reader may be unfamiliar with.

WILLIAM C. PHILLIPS

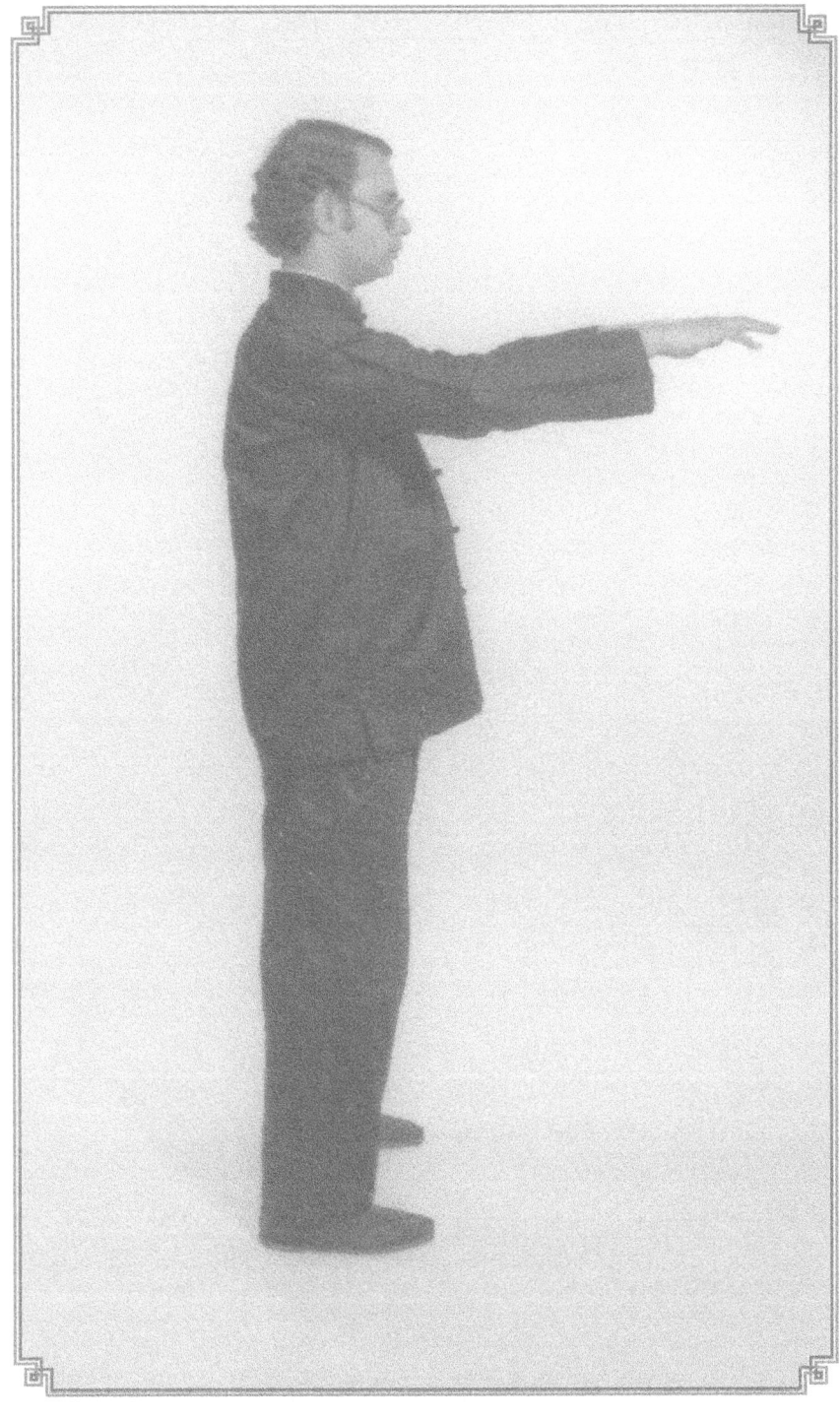

Chapter 1

The Preamble: or What Went Before

I started my training spending my high school years on the New Utrecht High School track team, primarily running cross country. I spent two and a half years practicing by running seven miles a day, five days a week – Monday to Friday, forty weeks a year – to run 2¼ miles at cross country track meets on selected Saturdays, at Van Cortlandt Park, in the fall. In spite of the practice, I was the slowest runner on my team and often fell over the finish line exhausted and coughing blood. I also occasionally participated in regular track meets, as a leg in the one- and two-mile relays, and running the mile (4:45 was my best time), half-mile (2:07), and quarter-mile (55.9 seconds, though any time under 60.0 seconds in the quarter was a victory over myself). I was really not a very good runner, but I had a great coach, Jackson Browne, who was endlessly patient with my efforts. I add this to my story because I think that those efforts caused me to start shaping my body, and led to my ability to stay the course, as I continued to stress muscles, breath, and stamina, in judo, ju jitsu, karate, and finally and ever after, in T'ai Chi.

At length, I graduated. Or maybe not at length, as I graduated in January of 1964, just days before my seventeenth birthday and a semester ahead of most of my classmates, and went on to college. My college choice set me on the path of the rest of my life, though it did not seem so at the time. That choice was Staten Island

Community College. It was located at 50 Bay Street, 28 Bay Street, and the 5th floor of 350 Saint Marks Place. It was a college around the "quad" of a municipal parking lot. At the end of my time there they took over the "Academy Building" and eventually moved into the "new" campus, alongside the Staten Island Expressway, and, when that got old, long after I graduated, finally into some new construction at the old campus of Willowbrook.

It would have made sense to go to Kingsborough Community College (KCC), which was in my own borough and where I later taught, but if I had gone to KCC, there would probably be no story to tell, and so I am glad I did not.

While studying as a liberal arts major in Staten Island in the fall of '64, a house plan was formed and I was invited to become a charter member. I declined, as my plate was full. I was on the school newspaper, the student court, and the student senate. Also, I was doing my best to keep my grades up.

But the house plan brothers seemed to be having a great time, throwing parties and meeting women. So, in the spring of 1965, I became a member of the first pledge class of Dolphin House, Staten Island Community College. A house plan is a fraternity on the cheap without Greek letters. Its house, apartment really, was at 1113 Avenue J, in Brooklyn, on the second story, in the front, over a Johns Bargain Store. The building is still there as of this writing. Our landlord, or sublessor, as he did not own the building, also at the same address, was Midwood Judo Center. The owner of the Dojo, Sensei Stan Israel, offered the members of Dolphin House a reduced rate for classes in ju jitsu and judo. Again, I didn't join in that first group. I thought I was a tough guy and could take care of myself.

The members who did join had so much fun throwing each other with hip throw (o goshi) and shoulder throw (ippon seoi nage) into the sofas on Friday nights before parties. I joined in the second group.

So, in September of 1965, I took the step that changed the

rest of my life: I joined the Midwood Judo Center. I learned about technical proficiency at the hands of my smaller and more innocent looking classmates, and that I was not so tough after all. My housemates all eventually stopped training, and I, alone of them all, remained. But here I get a little ahead of myself.

Getting a little ahead of the story, but necessary to relate was my mindset, then and after. I missed the sexual revolution and the drug revolution and even the political struggles of the '60s. I was occupied with four things, training in martial arts and teaching them, going to school, and going to work.

Once when I arrived at Brooklyn College for a class I had to step over protesters. I was not going to let them stop me from getting an education.

I missed Woodstock. A friend invited me to go with him, but I had to go to work and train that weekend, like every other. I drove a cab for a while in 1968 out of a barn on 18th Avenue in Brooklyn after work on nights when I did not train. I drove because becoming a new teacher was not a good way to become affluent or even pay the bills.

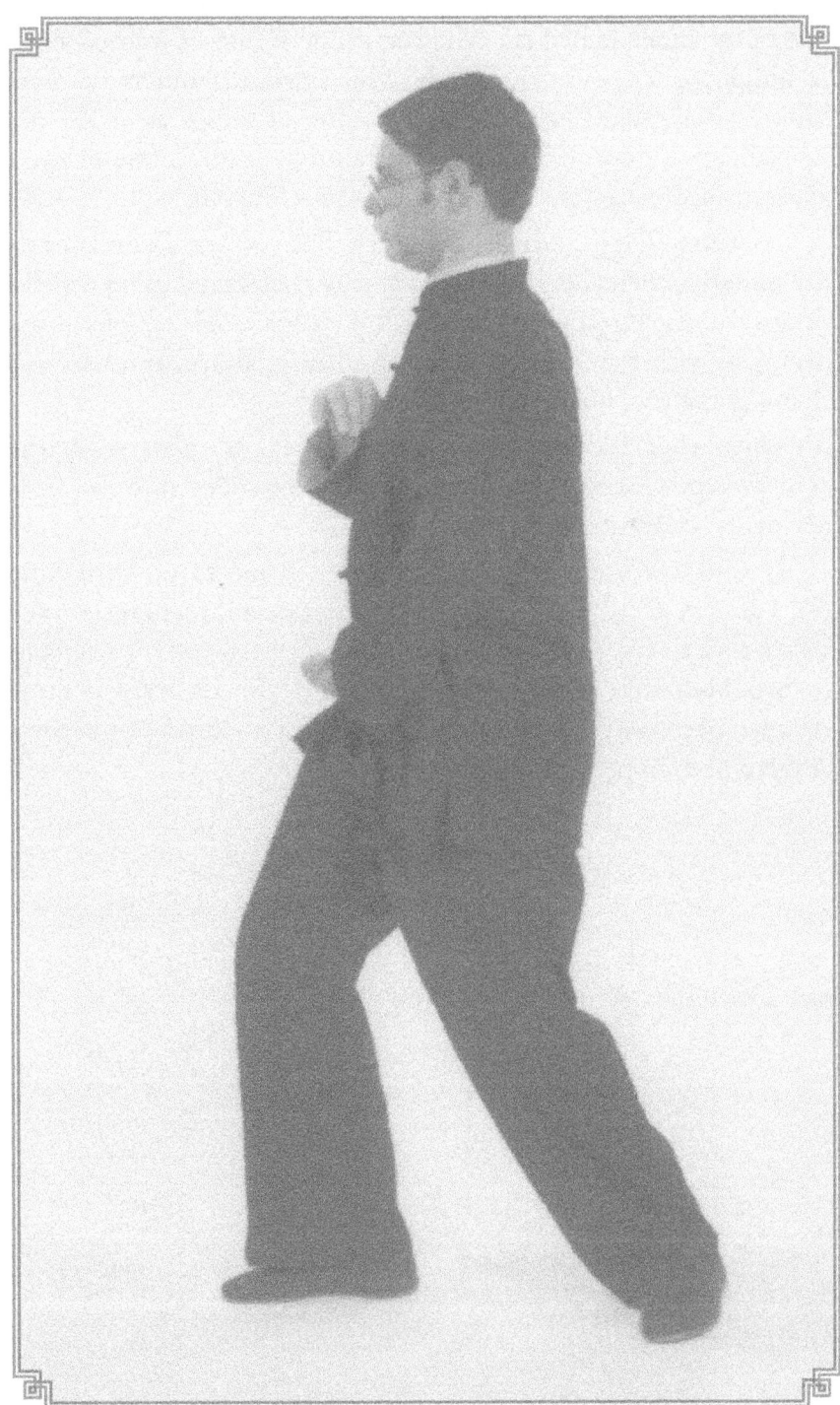

Chapter 2

Ju Jitsu, Judo and Karate, and How I Learned About T'ai Chi

After an indifferent start, I failed my yellow belt test. I never failed another martial arts test again. With that humiliation to motivate me, I started working very hard, training long hours, and making quick progress. I made brown belt, nikkyu, in judo (United States Judo Association, USJA) and ju jitsu in February of 1967. I made shodan in ju jitsu in February of 1969.

In 1967, I started karate under a couple of students of Herman Kauz. Since our ju jitsu included punching, kicking blocking, and sparring, I was well prepared for the karate but I was deficient in kata. Most of my training involved going over basics, correcting me for Shotokan methods, and learning kata; class typically finished up with sparring. I think I was moved along quickly in Shotokan, because I had done a lot of sparring in ju jitsu. Even as a Shotokan white belt, I could give my teachers a run for their money when we sparred.

I also started T'ai Chi in February of 1967 with Stan Israel in a room behind the Midwood dojo after class.

Ego Lesson

When I joined Stanley's school I had many lessons to learn, and my classmates were sometimes my teachers.

I remember that one of the most important lessons I learned was about ego. I learned it in judo. You could also say that the lesson was about technical proficiency. Fortunately, I learned it when I was a beginner. Back when I was a white belt, I rolled my gi (judo uniform) and put my white belt around it, swung it over my shoulder and strutted and swaggered off to judo class. After all, I had been a tough guy in junior high school and in high school. When I was a yellow belt and then when I added green tips to the yellow belt, I did the same. However, at green belt, I played judo against a smallish kid who did not look like much of a fighter or at all like a tough guy but had a brown belt. He threw me all over the place. Every time I got up, he threw me down again. Finally, after an hour or so, or maybe it just felt that way, I was too exhausted to get up and stayed down. All my ferocity and previous fighting skills were no help. After that incident, I would roll up my belt, put it into my gi, roll my gi, and put it into a blue plastic utility bag and go walking, meekly but eagerly, off to class.

The lesson was that being a tough guy does not mean you are technically proficient, a good fighter. What it does mean is that you fought and beat other people who were worse fighters. I was not technically proficient, but have been working on it ever since.

A Rivalry

I had an "epic" rivalry with one of my classmates: Marcel Weinberger. He had been in the first group to join Midwood Judo Center from my house plan. He was higher rank, having started in the first class, and he was bigger and stronger, but I was a bit faster. We sparred and played randori (sport judo) endlessly. We were about evenly matched and we competed with each other for roughly a year. Then he dropped out. I would like to tell you that I overcame and beat him. But that would not be true. Neither of us really ever got to be significantly better than the other. But he did drop out, and I remained, so I guess that is a victory of a sort.

Demonstrations

We did demonstrations for Stanley at various times and locations. I still have some fliers for those. I was trying hard, but definitely not up to the quality of a modern demonstration. I was only a green belt at first, and then a new brown belt. Yet, we introduced people to oriental martial arts. Who, today, would even look at such a demo except as a curiosity? Martial arts were new to people then, and so Stan got away with it.

By the way, I have some pictures of myself at demonstrations at that time, and my form really was not so good, especially when breaking boards. I think I may have just scared the boards into breaking.

Horse Stance

An interesting story of training with Stan comes to mind. Sometimes, starting when I was a green belt (yonkyu), during a Saturday class, he would leave us in horse stance for quite a long time. He would walk quietly behind us and correct us, sometimes by hitting us with a shinai, which made a loud noise but did not hurt much. Other times he would climb on our legs to make sure we were stable. Yes, all 200+ pounds of him standing on one of my legs, on the upper calf under the knee pit. Then he would continue to quietly walk behind us for a while. After he was confident (but wrong) that we were not sure where he was, he would step quietly off the mat, head for the instructor's dressing room, and get dressed. He would then proceed across the street to a kosher pizza place on the corner of East 12th Street and Avenue J for a scrambled egg and onion hero sandwich. Sandwich in hand, he would return, eat it quickly and quietly at his desk, then get into his gi and come back on the mat. He would then walk around behind us for a few more minutes as if he had never left, and then continue class. He thought we never knew he was gone, but we knew. As soon as he left, we would start to talk and adjust our stances if we were tired. Some guys would quit the stance until his return, but some of us were committed to getting stronger and would stay in the stance, maybe breaking our stance for a few seconds to stop the pain for a bit and then return to it. It was our private joke, the "eat the sandwich horse stance."

A Lucky Break

I played a lot of sport judo. They say that you get one major injury for every year that you play, so I guess I was lucky because I played for several years and only got one major judo injury: a broken collarbone.

I was nikkyu (2nd brown), playing a visiting dan-ranked friend of Stanley's who had just won the black belt division of an open tournament. I was giving him a very hard time. He was throwing me, but he was working for it. I should add, in case you are curious, I was not throwing him. In his frustration with me, he threw me with a left side osoto gari and straight-armed me in the collarbone to break my balance. Then he fell on top of me, arm still locked straight against my collarbone. He broke my collarbone when we landed. Stanley blamed him because he "should have known better" than to do left sided techniques, and "should have known better" than to fall straight-armed into someone. But I had been giving him a rough time and brought it on myself. Also, I held on, trying to counter until the last second, so I was at least partly to blame for his loss of balance as well.

Thereon hangs a humorous story. After that rather painful event I was bundled up and taken to the emergency room at Coney Island Hospital in my gi. After a long stay in the waiting room, watching people who were cut and much worse off than I was, getting triaged and admitted ahead of me, I was finally admitted to the hospital and was seen by the medical professionals. They seemed to think they were social workers. This was the '60s, and the ER doctors had not heard of judo, or seen a judo gi before. They kept telling me to own up to what seemed obvious to them: that my girlfriend had thrown me out of bed in my pajamas, and that is how I broke my collarbone. When they got tired of my protests that it was a judo injury, finally, they gave up on their misplaced social work, and got around to doing their jobs. They taped me up, issued me some painkillers, and gave me back to Stanley so he could take me home.

It took me a couple of months to get back into working out, and it turned out that this was a very lucky break indeed. At that time I had dropped from full-time day school at Brooklyn College (matriculated) to night school (non-matriculated) and was eligible for the draft. I was soon (as soon as the college sent notice of my changed status) called for an interview by my draft board. At that interview I protested that I had a freshly broken collarbone, but to no avail. I received a notice of an army medical examination at Fort Hamilton pursuant to being drafted shortly thereafter.

I went to the medical examination and, among other things, was subjected to a psychological test. There were only two questions. First the doctor asked me my name. When I answered by giving it, he said, "No identity problems." Then he asked me if I wanted to go into the army. When I said "no", he listed my answer as "Normal." I asked him what he would have listed if I had said "yes"? He said without hesitation, "Volunteer." There were no wrong answers.

When I got to a doctor for an examination of my broken collarbone, he said "I will pass you, you will be fine. They won't call you up for a couple of weeks, and it will be healed enough by then." I persisted, with my accompanying doctors' notes about the bone, and at length I received a two-month deferment (1–Y). I have to wonder about the quality of stateside army medical care. In the military, doctor's notes seemed to trump the physical condition. It was only by my having proof that a civilian doctor thought I was unfit and would not be fit for a couple of months that got me the deferment, and not the broken collarbone, which was present to be examined at the physical.

So I knew that if I did not want to be drafted, I had better start looking into rematriculating and getting my draft status of 2-S back. They took more than two months to reclassify me, and lucky they did. I just made it back to matriculated status. If I hadn't my story might have ended right here.

A Big Surprise

One time when I was a nikkyu brown belt, there was this big guy, 6'10" tall, about 240 lb, who stopped by the Midwood Dojo. He was huge. He was smart. It was his idea to visit schools and play randori with the people he thought he might meet at the promotional tournament in Rockville Center, later in the year. To perform well at the promotional, and thereby get a judo promotion, he wanted to know how his potential opponents played and what to expect. Stan thought the guy was playing to lose and learn at Midwood Dojo.

His strategy worked with me. I played him full out. That night I beat him good. I used my osoto gari and used it to set up my ippon seoi nage, or in English, I used my major outer reap throw and used it to set up (by faking for it) my shoulder throw. I beat him easily, maybe too easily. I did not think about things like that in those days. I was proud of the fact that I held up the school's honor in playing a visiting brown belt and winning, and a brown belt so much bigger than me at that. I learned something too: my tai otoshi was not working on him, nor my tomoe nage. In tai otoshi, a turn around tripping over the leg throw, I just could not get his balance. I would be fully turned, and just be hanging off his gi. In tomoe nage, a sit down and pull him over my extended leg throw, he was just too big. His feet were still on the mat when I was on the ground with my foot firmly planted in his stomach, so I just could not lift him. Stanley thought my ippon was the better of what worked and suggested that I work on it for the tournament. Stanley also suspected the osoto gari would not work. He thought the guy was falling for it to give me some false confidence for the tournament, something to try on him that he could easily defeat. So, figuring that I would meet him at the promotional, I trained ippon seoi nage, and trained it, and trained it, until my entry for the throw was smooth and as quick as the blink of an eye.

Sure enough, we met at the promotional, which is one of the few things I have on a bit of film. I had less trouble getting in on him than I had had at the school. In fact, I had no trouble at all. The training was working, or so I thought for an instant. I then realized that his strategy was not about keeping me out, it was about letting me in. It was also about using his size to stretch out over me as I pulled his torso, and then dropping down behind me and going for the choke hold.

When I was finished pulling, he still had his feet on the ground. He dropped to the mat behind me, pulled me over backwards, and tried to choke me out. I resisted, and the Japanese referee shouted, "Mate", and we stopped and got up. Having been caught by him dropping behind me, I should have caught on that he had worked out this strategy to beat me if I continued. I did not figure it out. I just tried harder and faster and got the same result the second time. This time he put his legs around my waist and pulled, trying to stretch me out as he tried to choke me, but I was pretty skilled at avoiding chokes. "Mate", the referee said forcefully, and we got up and continued playing.

Finally, since it was the only technique I had trained for this tournament, I gave it one more try. I should say here that since I had not trained anything else for this event, if it did not work, and I was still on my feet, I would have reached into my bag of other tricks, things which I had not worked on, not polished, for the promotional tournament.

However, this was not to be. I went in so very quickly and pulled with everything I had. My shoulder was almost to the ground and I thought I had him for sure. But as I looked between my legs, I saw that with my shoulder inches above the mat, and his shoulder inches above mine, his feet were still firmly on the ground behind me.

Oops. At that oops moment I realized that he had me. He sat down, wrapped his legs around my belly, stretched me out and choked me. This time, with two fresh lessons on how I evaded chokes, he choked me and I had to surrender or be put to sleep. I slapped out.

I was clearly the aggressor in the match, the only one with any offense, but I still lost. There were a couple of lessons for me in that match: First, the aggressive player may not be the winner and, second, don't tip your hand at the dojo, you may need your stuff for the main event.

Artie Brown

As time went on and the training continued, I found I gradually improved and could take care of business a lot more easily, if called upon to do so.

One day a new student showed up. Artie Brown had earned a nikkyu under Shina Sensei, on Bay Parkway. He told me that he had learned a lot and done well over there. He said he was pretty good and wanted to play randori to show me. I told him that I did not think I was that good. He wanted to play me anyway. As he was a new classmate, and we would be playing sooner or later, I said yes, and we played that Saturday afternoon.

Much to the surprise of both of us, I threw him, repeatedly, with multiple techniques. He did not throw me at all. I think his ego was wonderful, because when we were done, he told me that I must be very good because I was better than he was. I do not know if I believed I was really that good a player, or that I was just better than he was, which is what the evidence was showing me. After all, having been tossed around like a rag doll by Stan I was not one to really believe that I was particularly good. To this day I do not think of myself as really good at anything, but I know a lot of people who are worse than I am at a bunch of stuff.

Artie and I became friends and randori partners, as well as tournament buddies for a couple of years after that. He also joined Noguchi's training class and got thrown all over the mat with the rest of us. This gave us all our shot at becoming good together.

One story of those days comes to mind. It speaks to how busy and how active I was. One weekend in August I was invited by a friend to go to Woodstock for a rock and roll event (the famous event). I could not. On Friday I worked until midnight, on Saturday I trained from 10:00 AM until 3:00 PM and on the Sunday we (Artie and I and a girl named Renee) went to a tournament in Manhattan, at the 92nd Street Y. It was my bad luck to meet the under black belt division winner in the first round. My stuff was not working. He had counters to everything. After a couple of minutes of feints, he figured me out and threw me with a tomonage (he stuck a foot in my belly and sat down, over I went.) Artie won his first match with a makikomi (any throw, I do not remember which he used that goes to matwork, you throw and then drop on your opponent, and land in a grappling technique, kesagatame). He then choked his opponent out. He lost in a later round, I do not remember the details. That event was particularly memorable because it was my first experience as an official. When I lost, I was tapped to be a timekeeper and got to sit at the officials' table.

Noguchi

Taizo Noguchi was the 1967 All Japan Collegiate Judo Champion In 1968, when Noguchi was in New York City looking for a place to train, Stanley invited him to his class. Stanley had about thirty paying students before the night Noguchi joined us. Noguchi played randori with all of us that first night. Only a few of us returned, only those with brown belts, and not even all of them.

I played Noguchi early on in the class. It was a barrage of osoto gari, tai otoshi, ippon seoi nage, harai and hane goshi, foot sweeps, and more that I cannot remember. All this time I was trying my best to throw him. I had no luck and no skill that I had could do it either. Anyway, about 20 minutes into this barrage of throw after throw, I was thoroughly beaten and completely exhausted. When I could no longer rise to my feet quickly enough to suit him, he allowed me to bow out and went on to select his next victim. As I wanted to learn I, did not get dressed and leave, as did those of my classmates whom Noguchi had worked over before me. I stayed around to watch the rest of my class try against him.

One of my classmates towards the end of the line, who played Noguchi some time after I did, was this big guy, 6'2" or 6'3" and 250 lb or more of muscle. He was another of Stan's brown belts, about as good as I was, but a lot bigger, and a lot better muscled.

After throwing him with all his usual throws, Noguchi picked him up and threw him in a tremendous kata guruma, (shoulder wheel throw). My classmate went about eight feet in the air – high, that is – and maybe thirty feet down the mat. Now I did shoulder wheel throw myself, and no one went more than just up, over my shoulders, and down, maybe five feet up (to my shoulders) and three feet forward (to my right). So I was amazed. Just wowed. I had never seen the throw done like that, effortlessly, like Noguchi was tossing a feather pillow. My jaw dropped, I was stunned at the power of the move. In my awe, a mistake, I whistled. (In those days when you saw someone or something amazing, you may have done that, kind of like Humphrey Bogart in the movie Casablanca.) Noguchi, hearing me, turned his head towards me, like a swiveling tank turret, slow and steady, until he was looking directly at me through squinty eyes. He said, "No... Whisoo! You! ...No Whisoo!" He then swiveled his tank turret head slowly back to straight ahead.

A few seconds later, he threw the guy again, the same

incredible throw. My classmate spent an impossibly long, very, very long, time in midair. Then he fell, this time heavily, on the mat. I was again stunned at the power of the move. And then, in my awe, another foolish mistake, again, I whistled. I involuntarily whistled without thinking, and as soon as I emitted that long slow whistle, I knew it was a big mistake. I felt like a man who had just fallen off a cliff, thinking "Oh My God!" all the way down. Noguchi slowly turned his expressionless face to me. Then, he fixed me with a long and intensely dirty look. After looking at me for a few seconds, Noguchi started for me, hissing, "I said, You. No. Whisoo."

Stanley saved my life that day. He got between us and said, "Stupid American, he does not know any better." (Yes, he said "does not" so Noguchi would understand with his Japanese–English language skills, which were not that strong yet.). After a bit, Noguchi relented. Stanley thereby talked him out of tearing me apart and saved me grief, a pounding into the mat, and perhaps my life.

While this was going on, the guy Noguchi had thrown got up off the mat, and saw an opportunity in what was happening with me. Though he was not dismissed, though he did not bow out from playing randori with Noguchi, he bowed off the mat and went to the dressing room. He got changed, and left. He was never seen at Midwood Dojo again.

When Noguchi turned back to continue playing randori, he saw that his partner of the moment was gone. Without saying anything about this new disrespect, he selected another student and continued until he had played every one. After that class only a handful of us returned for these thrashings, and more importantly, to learn from Noguchi.

When Noguchi arrived, traditional learning stopped, and training, real training, started. With Noguchi, we would bow in and do some warm ups, including calisthenics. Then we would do ouchi komi, or in and out exercise, for throwing. (In ouchi komi exercise you do not actually throw the person you are working with, you just rapidly go in for the throw, break balance and stop and pop back out, then it is your partner's turn.) Then came some throw for throw exercises. One person throws the other, then the uke (person who is thrown) gets to become the torre (one who does the throwing). After an hour or so of these preliminaries came the main event: randori.

Noguchi was in one ring (one area on one side of the mat), Stanley was in the other. Randori, or sport judo, was played for the rest of the class. They each worked the class, which was not very big, just the three, four or five of us, whoever had shown up that night. They played us until we dropped (about half an hour apiece). When we had played one of them, we would queue up for the other one. When they were finished with us, they played each other for half an hour or so.

Stan was T'ai Chi good by then, but Noguchi could throw Stanley anyway. He often caught Stanley in a tai otoshi, osoto gari, ouchi or kouchi gari, or a foot sweep. Occasionally, not often, Noguchi would uproot Stanley and throw him with a high shoulder throw (ippon seoi nage). Stanley would go up, vertically, high in the air, above Noguchi, and then Stanley would seem to hesitate, suspended in air for a long second, and then come crashing down with a resounding thud that made the room shake to its foundations. Stan was soft and difficult to throw, unlike the rest of us. But when Noguchi threw Stanley high he landed like an earthquake, with the windows rattling and the floor reverberating.

After that we changed out of our gis and into street clothes. Noguchi then jogged up Avenue J and Bay Parkway to the Belt Parkway and along the belt to the Verrazano–Narrows Bridge. Stanley drove with us alongside Noguchi on the streets, and alongside him in the right lane with flashers on the Belt. Then we drove with him over the bridge and left him to jog up Bay Street and down Richmond Terrace to his apartment. For a job, Noguchi unloaded trucks at a supermarket all day (8:00 AM–4:00 PM). Then he came to class and played randori. Then he ran. Wow, just wow. Running as he did would be an incredible feat, even if he had not unloaded trucks all day and then played randori for hours. Deflecting my amazement, he said that to get on the judo team at his college, Waseda, (where Shina Sensei had gone to school, as well) you had to do 100 push–ups, 100 sit–ups, and 100 knee bends, without a break, just to be considered. He was in great shape, incredibly great shape. Working with him gradually put us into the best shape of our lives, though not in comparison to Noguchi.

After seeing Noguchi safely to Bay Street, Staten Island, Stanley and I would sometimes go to Chinatown to eat. More on that below.

Of course, we went with the New York team to the 1969 Amateur Athletic Union (AAU) Nationals. They were held in Chicago that year. New York fielded quite a team, with Noguchi at the top of the ticket in the open weight division.

To get to the AAU Nationals, we flew, a bunch of us, in a jet together. I packed very light, in an 8 mm projector case. I have never packed so well since. I am sorry to this day that I packed so light that I did not take a camera. Stanley played in, and Noguchi won, the open weight championship. New Yorkers were winning everything. Stanley, however, did not win, though I do not remember how he did, or who he played.

The night before the finals, we went out to find Japanese food. As we arrived at each restaurant, Noguchi walked right through every place we were considering and into the back, to the kitchen, and looked it over. We walked out of several fancy Japanese restaurants that evening. We finally ended up in a seedy Japanese diner kind of place, where he approved of the kitchen.

In the end, New Yorkers won almost every division. Then they had a play-off of division winners for the grand champion of the event. The last match of the Nationals was Noguchi against Allen Coage, another New Yorker, who had won the heavyweight division.

In that final match for the grand championship, Noguchi broke Allen Coage's arm with a flying arm bar right before my eyes. I was sitting in the first row, right in front of that ring. Since they were both playing for NY, Noguchi had warned Coage not to grab high, but Coage had done it any way. Noguchi got a standing arm bar on him, and threw his body out to the side, completely horizontal, with an incredibly crisp snapping movement. They came down as a unit. Allen Coage's arm was broken. The match was over, Noguchi won.

At the end of the tournament, Noguchi was awarded a big trophy, it must have been six feet tall. On our way out at checkout from the Drake hotel, the big trophy was on the floor between us on the checkout line, Stan was in front of us. A girl came over and asked Noguchi if the trophy was his. He slyly said no, that he played Tennis. He then said it was mine. She gave me an adoring look. I had an awkward moment, I did not know what to say. I just pointed back at Noguchi, and smiled.

Shortly after, Noguchi went back to Japan to start a career as an executive in Supermarkets/retail food.

Fun with Stanley

Liking the experience of going to eat after dropping Noguchi, Stanley and I got in the habit of enjoying a night out in Chinatown, just the two of us. We continued going out once every week or two, until the end of Stanley's ownership of Midwood Judo Center.

Sometimes we would just eat, and I would be home between midnight and 1:00 AM. On our more extended evenings, we would go to Chinatown to watch a movie and then eat. We had to go to the movie first because the theaters in Chinatown closed around midnight. After eating we would call it a night and Stan would drive me home. On those nights I would arrive home much later. On occasion, we would go uptown and see another movie on 42nd

Street. At the time 42nd Street had a long row of theaters showing everything from first run to B movies: westerns, sci fi, and war pictures. I think I remember seeing *2001: The Space Odyssey*, *The Good, The Bad and The Ugly* as well as *Where Eagles Dare* with Stan, in midtown, in the middle of the night. Then it was back to Chinatown for a breakfast of some veggies and meat over rice, and then home. Stanley usually got me home by about 6:00 AM, barely in time to change and leave for work, without any sleep. Stan, of course, got to go to sleep, as he had no obligations in the mornings.

I would like to state right here that I do not/cannot do that anymore. These days I fall asleep between 9:00 PM and 11:00 PM if left to my own devices. Also, in those days I could eat 5000 plus calories a day and not gain an ounce of fat. My weight rose from 125 lb to 165 lb after I started my training. It was all muscle.

I Begin To Teach

Shortly after Noguchi left, I made shodan in ju jitsu. When that happened I started helping Stan teach, both inside the school and outside as well. I was given a Sunday Class of my own, where I collected the money, and had students uniquely mine as well as Stan's.

However, actually getting paid was another matter. We had a rather unusual arrangement for this class. I was supposed to get half the money, paid by the students whom I got to join my Sunday class. So, I started with a bunch of my friends, and gave Stan his half of the money. Then he started sending dojo students to the class. When I asked him for my half of that money, he always said to speak to his wife. When I asked her for the money she always said I had to speak to Stan. Ms. Israel was probably not in on it, just reluctant to disburse cash without Stan's say so. But Stan probably got a laugh out of it. Eventually, as will happen, all my friends dropped out and I taught yet another class free for

Stan. All the other classes I taught for Stan were considered to be my dojo service. Good students were expected to give back. I guess this one turned out to be my service as well. Though later, when I became a teacher in my own school, I paid my students for the teaching work that they did, as I did not want to subject my students to the more traditional method that I came up through.

I had been given two weeknight classes at Midwood Dojo as my school service. I had the early classes, 7:00 PM to 8:30 PM, then someone else got the later slot, 8:30 PM to 10:00 PM, giving Stan the night off. Various people had the class after mine. For a while it was Rick Lenchus, of House of the Legend fame, then it was a Shotokan black belt I did not know, finally it was Herman Kauz.

I was also accompanying Stan to the YM/YWHA, on Linden Blvd. where we both put on gis and Stan sat and socialized with the parents while I taught the kids class. I did not have a car in those days so Stan drove. Later, when Stan joined the Correction Department, he left that class to me and I got paid for it. In fact, I may still have a pay stub from those days.

Herman Kauz at Midwood Dojo

Sensei Herman Kauz was a very qualified Shotokan sensei. He had been, for a while, the highest-ranking non–Japanese in Shotokan karate, as well as an Hawaiian state judo champion. He was studying T'ai Chi with Professor Cheng as well. After the six senior students, he was the next best at T'ai Chi.

While he was teaching Shotokan at Midwood Dojo, one of my ju jitsu students, who had an incredibly large ego and thought I was a wonderful teacher, made one of those "ultimate errors."

Now you have to understand, I knew I was no match for Herman; I also knew that this kid was no match for me. The kid, a green belt, should have known that as well, but he thought I had taught him so well, he could defeat a man who could easily defeat me. To top it off, the kid was about five feet tall, to Herman's six feet something.

He challenged Herman to spar. Herman accepted. Well, the sparring was kind of one sided, with Herman raising welts all over the kid's chest. Herman would give the kid a few seconds to respond, or perhaps to register that he'd been hit. When no response was forthcoming, Herman would just hit him again. Every time Herman punched or kicked his chest, another welt would appear. Eventually, the kid knew he had had enough and bowed off.

I was a pale green color during this whole encounter. When it was over, Herman turned to look at me, and all I could do was get out a muffled, "I did not send him, it was his own idea." I thank God and Herman that he took my word for it, and did not challenge me. This was because the kid had committed a severe breach of etiquette, and I, as his teacher, was responsible. If I had known in advance what the kid had in mind, I would have been able to stop him. I was very fortunate that Herman looked at me and saw that I was sincere and said it was OK. That was the end of that embarrassing episode.

I Begin Karate

January 1967 I started karate under a couple of dan ranked (black belt) students of Herman Kauz. They corrected me to Shotokan ways, as my techniques were quite effective, but definitely not Shotokan. Also, and more importantly, I had to learn the kata. After learning the kata, I had to perform them well.

I was very good at sparring, as that had been part of the ju jitsu I had learned. With amazing quickness, I was promoted to shodan, first-degree black belt, in February 1969. In part my quick rise had to do, I think, with the fact that they would not let me wear my ju jitsu rank on the mat. So here was this white belt that was going toe to toe with the senseis of the class. At any rate, I saw making dan rank as a license to teach, and that is just what I did.

I Get Interested in the Soft, Moving Towards T'ai Chi

An interesting happening in the late '60s was the visit of a high-ranking (9th dan) judo practitioner from Japan to the McBurney YMCA, in Manhattan. This little old man, wearing a red belt, was about 5'4" tall, and about 140 lb. He came with a taller and stockier assistant, wearing a red-and-white striped belt. They went through an impressive demonstration. The red belt threw his assistant with all kinds of throws, most I had seen before, and some that I had never seen. The assistant could not throw the red belt, at all. As they were concluding, a young American nidan or sandan, maybe 6'4" and 250 lb stood up and challenged the old man. They played randori. The old ninth dan let the youngster attack. Though tall and strong, the younger man just could not throw the older man. He had no more success than the red-and-white striped belt had. The American went in for a tai otoshi, and the red belt just stood there, as if he were a post stuck in the ground. The young man went in for a hip throw, and the elder man went over, landed on his feet, facing, and then slid under and did a sumi gaeshi to the American. He continued to throw him all over the place as he had thrown his assistant. This demonstration of an older gentleman easily defeating a strong youngster, solidified my wish to want to study with Professor Cheng. There were techniques of softness out there so that strength and youth may be overcome.

Earlier in 1966, Stan had introduced me to Robert W. Smith's book, *Secrets of Shao Lin Temple Boxing*. I was enthralled with the internal. So in February of 1967, Stan invited me to stay after class on Saturdays and learn T'ai Chi Ch'uan privately. That was the start of my T'ai Chi training, which would last for three years under Stanley. First he taught me the form, and then push hands. After that, he would correct my T'ai Chi form, and play push hands with me, decorating the wall with me really, as he pushed me repeatedly for an hour and more at a time, late on Saturday afternoons. We trained after ju jitsu class, in a back room that he had rented to an organization that rarely used it. It was empty late on Saturday afternoons, at least when we trained there. This additional training was after a couple of hours which included warm ups, a lesson, punching and kicking, ouchi komi (in and out for throwing exercise), throw for throw exercise, horse stance, randori, and sparring in the regular Saturday class.

Stan often talked of a little old man in Chinatown who could do amazing things in Chinese medicine (such as heal allergies; I had been taking shots and pills, which either did not work, or worked temporarily, since I was a kid). This old man also did T'ai Chi, which included throwing Stan around.

Now throwing Stan around was a feat I had only seen done by one person, our judo instructor, Taizo Noguchi. He was youthful, fast, powerful, and muscled beyond belief. So how could a little 70 something year old man in Chinatown be able to do the same thing to Stan? (When I later joined the school I saw that he did it much more regularly than Noguchi ever had; he pushed Stan pretty much at will.)

That little old man was the T'ai Chi master, Professor Cheng Man-Ch'ing. He was like the hero in some martial arts movie, except in real life. Stanley always said to me, "One of these days I will take you to meet, study with, and get some medicine from this man, Professor Cheng." But while whetting my appetite with many amazing stories about Professor Cheng, Stan was not forthcoming about the whereabouts of the teacher, and it never seemed to be the right time for Stanley to take me to meet the Professor.

Since Stan said it was "too complicated" to bring me to Professor Cheng, if I had waited for Stanley's introduction, my story would end right about here.

We Get a Dose of Spirit

Stanley got wind of some Tibetan Lamas coming to New Jersey, and we made arrangements to go and see them and listen to them give a talk. My wife at the time (now ex) could not understand this. She had never heard of Tibetan Lamas and thought we were going to see some of the South American kind, llamas, just from Tibet. She could not figure out why we wanted to go to a house in New Jersey and not to a zoo to see them. When I said they were giving a talk, she thought I had lost my cookies, so to speak. When I came back and said I had them on tape, she said she wanted to hear them and asked if they were like Mister Ed. I thought this was hilarious. She just did not know, and when I played the tape, she finally understood.

My Time at Midwood Dojo Comes to a Close

At length, it was time for Stan to move on with his life, and he got a job with the Corrections Department of the City of New York as a prison guard. Once that happened, he could not be at Midwood Dojo and so he had to sell it. At length, he sold it to Charlie Musante.

I was finally put on salary: $5.00 a class. Charlie ran the school with a woman named Veronica. It sounded like I would be able to stay, even in Stan's absence, but Sensei Musante wanted to have final say on all promotions as this was his school. Stanley had not bothered me about stuff like this, he had not looked over my shoulder. Stan had left my under belt (less than brown and black belt ranks) promotions to me. I was upset about this, feeling that as the teacher of the students I should be the one in charge of promotions. I had no problem with Charlie coming to the tests, and even putting his two cents in. I had a problem giving tests and then submitting the results to him to decide, considering that he was not even there for the tests. Yet it was his school, and he wanted to decide.

So, over this disagreement in the administration of promotions,

I left Charlie, Veronica and Midwood Dojo. I went on to sublet space for my own classes from a friend and T'ai Chi classmate, Lenny Antonucci, at his place on 20th Avenue and 71st Street (7108 - 20th Avenue). This was my first dojo space on my own, at least on Monday and Wednesday nights. And I could run my own promotion examinations, without anyone looking over my shoulder.

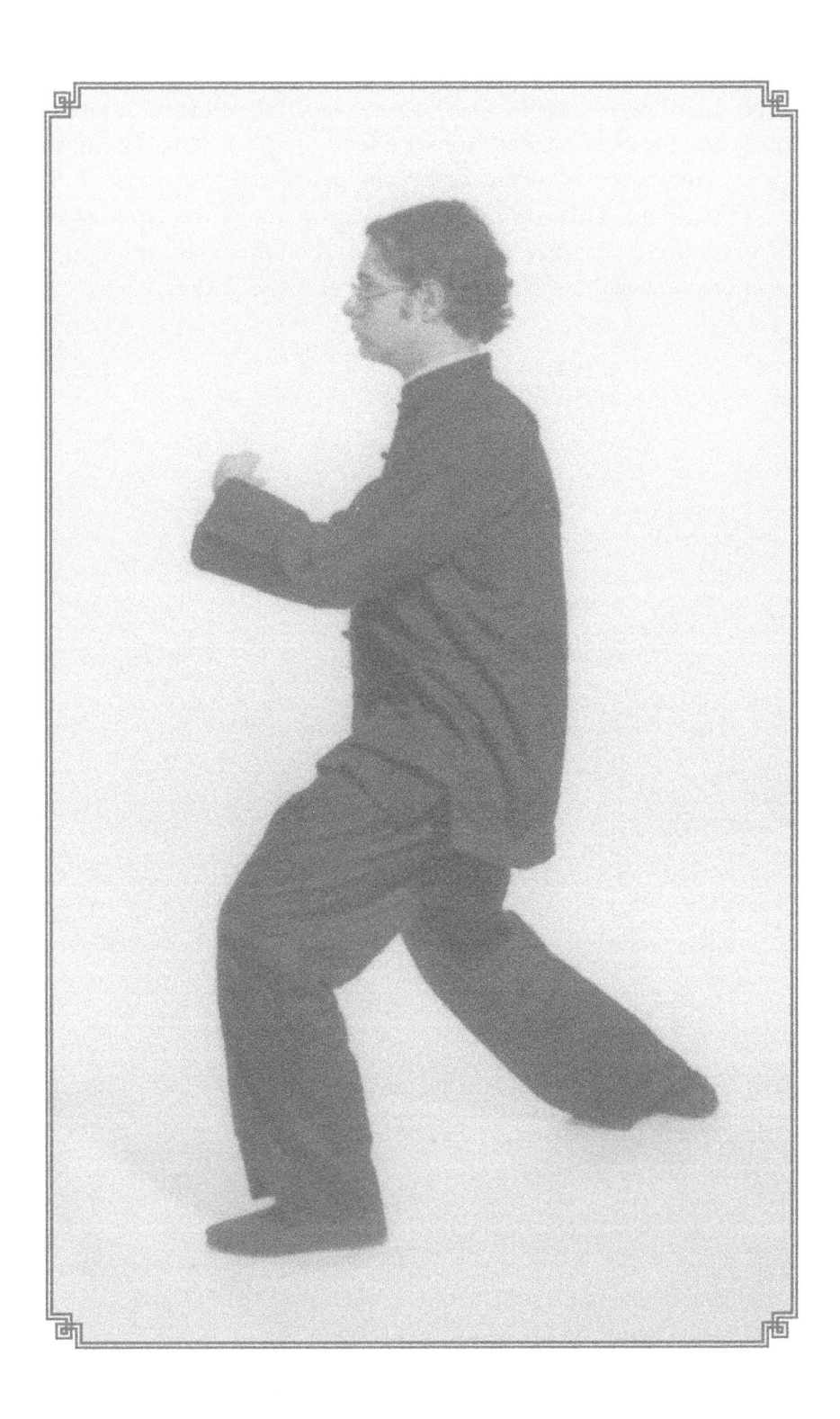

Chapter 3

Stanley Israel at Midwood Dojo

I need to pause here, to digress, and discuss Stanley Israel more fully in the context of the story. I wish to write a few words about the complex man who was Stanley Israel. I knew Stanley Israel since 1965, the longest of any of the people I am writing about. He was my house plan's landlord, my ju jitsu and judo teacher, as well my first T'ai Chi teacher, and a senior student of Professor Cheng, one of the senior six in New York. When I started to teach ju jitsu, he was my employer, then my classmate in Professor Cheng's school, and finally an unpaid co-teacher at Patience T'ai Chi.

He was one of my best friends for a long stretch of time. But Stanley was ... well, complicated, to say the least. Though he did some things that hurt, for example the pay issue in the Sunday class (when I was really poor and could have used the money), and never giving me a copy of my film (that story will come up in its place), I felt it was still well worth it to be his friend. What it cost me to be Stanley's friend were minor pin pricks compared to the fun and entertainment of hanging around with him.

Playing chopsticks

He was Stanley, and he had his ways. For example, there is the way he taught me to eat with chopsticks. Stanley would occasionally take us out to eat at a Chinese restaurant, usually after we did a demonstration for Midwood Dojo, his first school. He eventually owned three others, Bay Ridge Dojo, Kings Highway Dojo and Sheepshead Bay Dojo. At these Chinese banquets with us students, we all paid a share and each of us ate what he or she could eat from the communal dishes Stanley ordered. As a senior student of Stanley's I always sat at his side at these communal meals.

Stanley insisted that I eat with chopsticks, and if I tried to take the food with a fork, as I did at first, his chopsticks would, in a flash, swoop in and steal the food right off that fork. He was very good with those chopsticks. As a result, I paid my share but did not eat my share. So finally, after several of these meals, I learned the hard way. If I wanted to eat anything at these banquets, I had to eat with chopsticks. If I wanted to eat any reasonable amount of food, I had to learn to eat quickly and well with the sticks. So I picked up my chopsticks and started to try to use them. I found that he would let me eat as I struggled with the sticks, even if I used them as spears to get some food to my mouth. As I got better, I started to get to eat more food at these feasts, and I never looked back at a fork in a Chinese restaurant. I am sure Stanley got a laugh out of his method of teaching me. A tough love method for sure. He must have cared, as he did not do this to anyone else, just me.

This story is more fun in retrospect than it was at the time.

Friend and businessman

Stanley dealt more fairly with me than he dealt with others. I say that in spite of the pay issue. He offered to sell me Midwood Judo Center and its income for $3000. Then, when I could not raise the money, he sold the Dojo to Charlie Musante, for $6000.

While Stan was a business man, and a good one, he was more than just about the money. When he had the opportunity to train with the best, he took it, and money be damned. Noguchi was the

1967 All Japan Collegiate Judo Champion. As I related above, in 1968, Noguchi was here in New York City looking for a place to train. Stanley had Noguchi come to our school to teach and train judo, and lost many students who found the training too hard. He destroyed a good class. But in order to learn judo from a champion, Stanley was fine about losing his best-paying adult class. He never regretted the lost revenue, though it was his living, because he saw an opportunity for himself, and for us, to learn.

SECRETS, ALWAYS SECRETS

Stanley was secretive. Stanley had a most incredible root, he had one foot back, but not so far back you would notice it, yet you could not push him over it. Even Professor Cheng himself had commented positively about Stanley's skill. But Stan did not teach it to anyone, though you were welcome to feel it, especially while playing randori. He would bounce you off, and then throw you before you could recover your balance.

He also had the open snap strikes. Once I saw him do the soft style inside block and it became my signature move in later years. I asked him how he did that, and he would not answer. He merely said, "It's complicated." Then he walked away, down the mat to correct someone else.

But if Stanley had not shown the technique, I never would have known it was possible. So, thank you Stanley. Maybe he was teaching "zen" style, like with the chopsticks, and half the lesson was to take the move apart and figure it out. Well, that is just exactly what I did.

I figured that move out for myself, and did great things with that powerful technique in later years. I turned it over and did an open snap strike with my right hand, and it could be faster than the eye could follow if it was coming at you. It is powered through the legs and hips, and it is also how the fa chin, and the no-inch punch happen. It's the same principle.

But I did not learn them from Stanley. I learned them from two of my less favored teachers: trial and error.

Stan: The Story Gets Ahead of Itself, for a Reason

After an incident that happened at the Shr Jung, most of us left. We did not see each other for several years. One day some time later Stan showed up at Patience T'ai Chi. He started watching class. After a few weeks of this, he began coaching my students. After class, he would take me out and buy me a slice or two of pizza. Then he would drive me home in his Cadillac (In the healthy bad old days I would jog the ¾ mile, and later ½ mile, to my school to teach the classes). Stan had a car phone, long before ONSTAR, and our conversations were sometimes interrupted by calls. We talked about the old days, my student's prospects for tournaments, and whatever else came up.

Shortly after the start of his coming to my school on Thursday nights, I was placed on an extremely early session at work. Due to this I would leave Patience T'ai Chi promptly at 8:00 PM, having taught from 7:00 PM to 8:00 PM. Class was scheduled to go till 9:00 PM or later (as late as anyone would stay). Jimmy Leporati was in charge of the second hour. Stanley, who typically stopped by at about 7:30 PM or so, would sit and watch the conclusion of the form instruction.

Then, when the push hands instructions started, he would observe carefully, and coach. Stanley was an expert at push hands, beaten by no one except Professor Cheng. He coached with wisdom and good advice. He never gave bad advice to, or played games with, any of my students. At about that time, the students started going out to eat Chinese food at Ocean Palace Chinese Restaurant after class. When they went out to eat, sometime after 9:00 PM, he would join them and they had wonderful times talking and eating, sometimes practicing or demonstrating between the tables. I would join them when I did not have to be at work the next day (I was a school teacher and so there were many vacation days). Great wisdom, great philosophy and pretty good jokes were in abundance. A great time was had by all.

The reason

Stan never fooled around with any of my students with his advice. I say this because Stan was a kidder, as this story will indicate:

At Midwood Judo Center (his business, and his only one in my student days) there was no air conditioning, we only had open windows. One hot, humid summer Saturday, Artie Brown and I and a few of the other brown belt students were sitting around with him after class. We were still in our gis, cooling off at the desk, after an impossibly heavy, sweaty workout. It was just too hot to get dressed, as our sweat would not dry. So there we were, chewing the proverbial fat, and recuperating in the late afternoon.

As we sat at the desk, a man came bouncing up the stairs who wanted to study karate. Stan looked at us, winked, and began to wax poetic and hyper enthusiastic, which was not like Stan at all: "Yesss... a karate man would beat a judo man, a karate man would beat a ju jitsu man, a karate man would beat a kung fu man, a karate man would beat a savate man," and on and on and on. The guy ate it up. We were nodding our agreement with Stan on the outside, laughing on the inside, because we had never seen this side of Stan. Eventually, the man enthusiastically signed up and left. We waited for the man to go down the stairs, and then burst out in loud peals of laughter a minute after he had disappeared. We laughed, not because we agreed or disagreed with Stan, but because it was not Stan's way to be so enthusiastic. We enjoyed Stan doing a comedy show, apparently, just for us.

Somewhat later that afternoon, in came another potential customer. The guy said he wanted to study judo because he had heard that judo was the best martial art in the world. Stanley warmed to his topic and started off again saying that he could not agree more. He again went on to say that a judo man would beat a karate man, a judo man would beat a kung fu man, a judo man would beat a ju jitsu man, a judo man would beat a savate man, and on and on and on, with great enthusiasm. We were again cracking up with laughter on the inside even worse than before, as Stan was putting on a show. While the potential customer was in the room, we were mum, occasionally quietly nodding our heads in agreement with what Stan was saying. When he had signed up and left, all the way left, cleared the staircase and was in the street, we laughed out loud, long and hard, but just not so the potential customer could hear us. We hoped.

Stan had just enthusiastically endorsed both judo and karate as the best martial art, and we enjoyed that immensely.

Finally, as we were preparing to get up out of our chairs, change, and go home, yet one more seeker came up the creaky staircase. He wanted kung fu. We did not offer kung fu but Stan was on a roll, and he once again performed. At the end he had to admit that he did not offer what the man wanted. The man thanked Stan profusely for telling him the "truth" and went off in search of kung fu. We went in search of our composure, which was greatly missing after Stan's latest performance.

But ever after, if I hear of someone telling me what Stan told them, I take it with a grain of salt. Not because I think they are lying, but I do not know how Stan may have come to "tell" them. He may have been pulling their leg. Another consideration is that he also had a talent for letting a blind man go on being blind, through just not disagreeing. If a man is attached enough to an opinion, he would not try to disabuse him of it. If you wanted his opinion, he felt you should ask for it with your cup empty. If your cup is filled with an opinion in it, why waste that opinion? You cannot make this stuff up. What did Stanley really believe? I will let you wonder about that one.

Some other stories about Stanley.

A SHOT, NOT IN THE DARK

Then there was the time when he first became a Correction Officer, and insisted that he come up to my apartment at 8758 Bay Parkway, to shoot his .25 caliber pistol. I was terrified at the prospect. I was unable to dissuade him from his plan. At length, from the foot of my bed, he shot at a phone book he had placed on pillows at the head of my bed. Fortunately, in my fear, I had pestered him so much about being careful that he shot low and put the bullet into the bed itself. I had his bullet in my mattress for many years after. And I had a hole in my only queen bed sheet, or my bed shoot as I jokingly called it after that. I slept on that mattress until I got married and had to buy another bed.

DINNERS AND MOVIES

In the evenings, as I have already noted, Stanley and I often went out to eat and to the movies. I remember one Chinese New year when we started out at a movie at the Music Palace movie theater on the Bowery, and then went to eat. Next we watched lion dancing and firecrackers on Mott Street in the cold night. Then we went up town and saw a movie on 42nd street. After that we went back to Chinatown to eat at Sam Wo's at around 5:00 AM. They mopped the floors while we were eating, so we had to raise our feet off the floor so they could mop under our feet. Stan would point out all the well-known judo and karate people in the place. Did anyone in martial arts go to bed early? Apparently not, in those days. Then he drove me home, and went home himself. That morning I got home with a fever, just in time to call in sick, and then slept the day away. I remember being feverish and exhausted on at least one other Chinese New Year by the time we got to the movies on 42nd Street, but enjoyed the movies and the food any way.

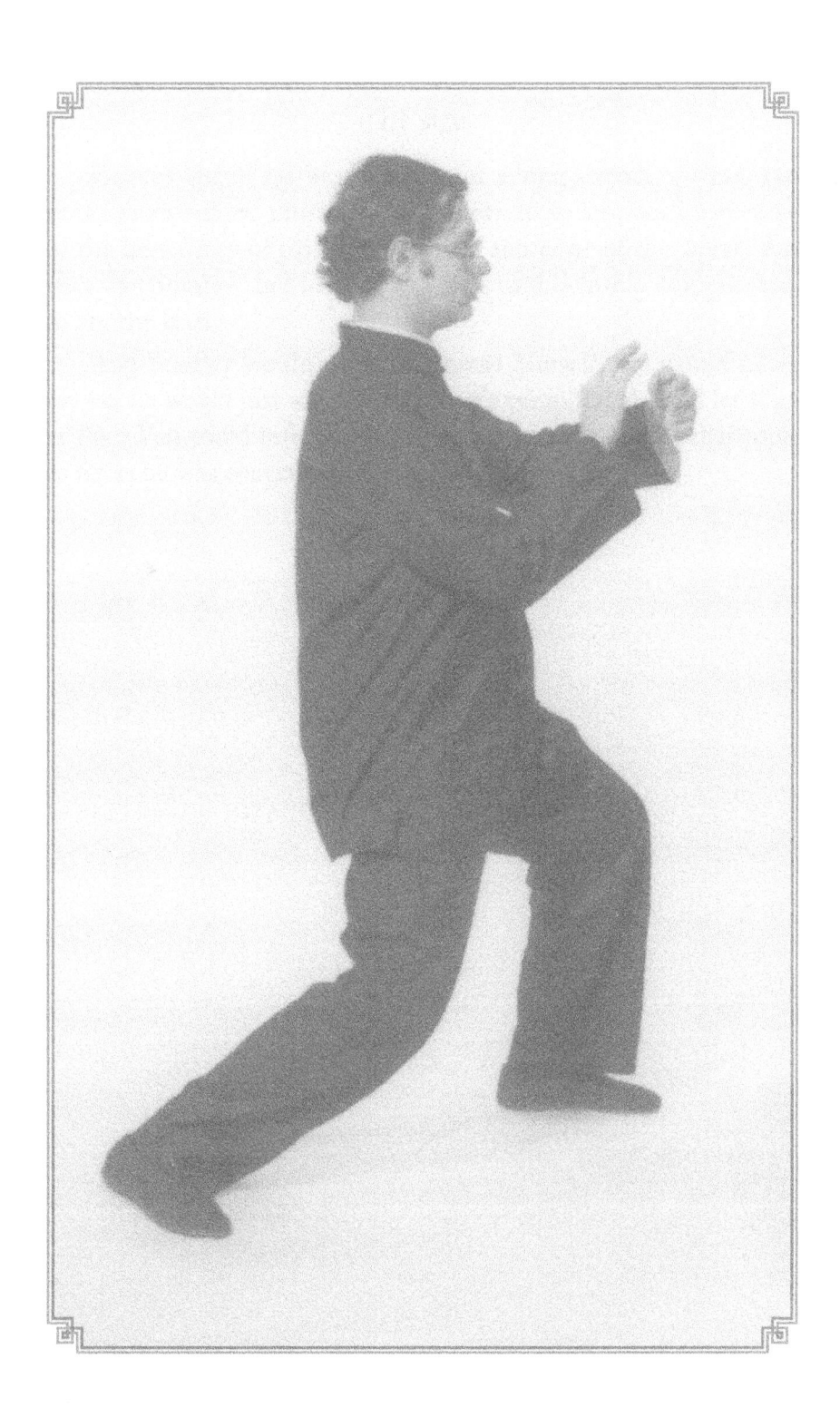

as well, and occasionally made additional corrections. When he watched me like that, I was proud and thought he could see that I was doing it well, though I presumed he did not know of my previous training. That was something I was sure that no one else in the class had: previous training. But pride is stiffness... (and I was quite stiff as it was).

This led to an embarrassing error on my part. Once, during class, while we were standing in White Crane Spreads Wings, waiting for Professor Cheng's correction, Professor put his hand on my raised arm and went to push it down. I was not sure what to do. I instinctively relaxed and let him push it down, then I started to resist, then I let it go again. In the end I resisted because I thought that was what he wanted. He looked at me, smiled and walked away. Later I asked a senior student what I should have done. He said I should have been as soft as I could be and let him move my arm as freely as I could. On hearing that, I was frustrated and embarrassed. I wanted to be seen as a good student. I had had a chance to do that by being totally as soft as I could be, and I had blown it. In retrospect, even my soft was not that soft in those days, though it was my first instinct to be as soft as I could. I must have seemed stiff, even in my softness and then totally stiff, as I offered resistance.

I had ch'i in my fingers early on, and Professor may have known it, just from looking at me. I was afraid to just speak up about it. Finally, I gathered up my courage and asked about it and was told by Professor that I was correct. I did have ch'i in my fingers. The trouble was that, while I had had it for weeks, when I spoke of it, I got so nervous that the feeling of it went away for quite a while. Eventually the experience of ch'i came back, and now I am talking about it and it is not in any danger of going away.

I LEARN HUMILITY AGAIN: A UNIQUE DEMOTION

In due time, the class I was in finished the form. We were the very last class that learned the new postures directly from Professor, where only he taught the new postures. We were also lucky to have him correct some of us on the older postures as well, as we promptly misinterpreted them soon after he taught them. After this, the entire class was "promoted" to being allowed to play push hands. With one exception.

Professor called me over and had some words for me in Chinese. The interpreter told me I was to do the form again. I did not have permission to play push hands, but was to start the form again the following week, with the next beginners' class. I did not understand it. I had three years of T'ai Chi with Stanley Israel before I ever got to Professor's class. I thought my form was clearly better than most of my classmates because I had those three years more experience and had practiced it at least twice daily since I started. The new pieces were not new to me. I thought I was being demoted, held back. I felt humiliated. My ego was instantly deflated. But I did not show it. I was embarrassed, as I had thought I was better than my classmates, and now the implication was that I was worse. I quietly did as I was told.

Yep, I thought, I really did blow it when I was not relaxed when he pushed on my arm. But later I came to understand that he "demoted" me because he liked my form (or me?) and wanted to give me an opportunity to continue to improve before going on to push hands. Thus, much later, I was aware that I had come to his notice in a good way, in spite of my pride, my embarrassment, and my stiffness.

Professor Cheng had less to do with that class, as at that time the senior students were now permitted to teach the new pieces. And so, the senior students ran the entire class. But the

Professor came by and watched the class from time to time. He continued to correct me, and some of the others as well, in that class.

It was at this time, when I stayed late after my class, that I got to watch push hands, sword form, and dueling. I knew that you could not do them until the form was finished. I knew that you had to be in push hands for a time as well before you could be promoted to learning sword form, then you could get permission to duel. I knew that these were the advanced trainings. I put them in order as I saw them. Push hands was unarmed, and it is what we got permission to do after we finished the form, so it was the next skill. So push hands did not appear, to my beginner's mind, to be that advanced. The order seemed to be: form, push hands, sword form, then sword dueling. I thought that the dueling was the most advanced thing I was seeing. I could not wait to get to dueling. When I got permission to film, I filmed that the most. If I had it to do again, I would have spent a lot more time filming push hands.

Ahh. The mistakes we make, when we base our actions on our youthful judgments.

After the end of my second form class, I was given conditional permission to go on to push hands. My classmates had gotten an unlimited permission to join in push hands with any one they wanted. They did not have any supervision beyond a senior student keeping an eye on the freestyle push hands wall, so that class did not get out of hand. After going through the form twice, I only received permission to learn and practice push hands under a mentor. Unlike any one else in my class, I still only half graduated from form, even after two classes. They all had permission to play free style push hands with everyone. I could play, but I could not play with just anyone. Again, Professor took an interest in seeing that I was learning, and again I interpreted it as a non–promotion, wondering what I might have done wrong. No one else that I saw got that kind of treatment.

Professor Cheng had asked Mort Raphael to mentor me, teach me, and keep an eye on me.

It was the beginning of a friendship, and also of a very frustrating time for me, and for Mort. Mort tried to teach me to relax, and to teach me the difference between relax and collapse. Because of my youth and success with my muscles in the martial arts, I was not a very good student of relax. So Mort designed exercises to help me, and he tweaked my nose with frustration when I learned the exercise, but not the lesson the exercise was intended to teach. I was pretty dense, but both Mort and I, we persisted, and so here I am today writing this book. Also, because of Mort's example, I learned how to better design exercises to showcase the principles that I wanted to get across. I do this today when I am teaching, but I am getting ahead of myself, ahead of this book.

People have asked me why I was not taught fighting applications. I want to say, right here, in case it is not obvious. While I was a dan rank (black belt) when I arrived in Professor Cheng's school, I was young, strong, and very successful with strong techniques. I was stiff, and way too much of a beginner, though I did not know it, to be taught applications. However, I had faith in Professor and was happy to learn whatever Professor wanted to teach. I understand now that I was way too stiff and strong. Professor filled my cup from the bottom up, with what I had to learn first.

If I had been taught applications, and learned them the only way I could have understood them then, in a very stiff way, and thought I had them, I would have missed the beauty and elegance of his art. I would have missed the whole point of it. And, though I thought I was kind of relaxed and soft, Mort started me on the path that would lead to real relaxation and softness. It was a path that led over a long and bumpy road.

Professor Sees My Future

I started attending Professor Cheng's lecture class that was held on Fridays (more on that later). Since I was a high school teacher and was home early, I picked up my steady date downtown. She worked for a courier outfit in the financial district. After she finished her days' work, I picked her up in my car and we then went to the T'ai Chi Association. While I attended the class, she waited for me, sitting on a comfortable green chair in the anteroom, reading. I used to tease her—that she had a black belt in watching, though she read a book and did not watch. When the class was over, and I was ready, we would go out to eat in Chinatown. We ate at Sum Hey Rice shop, on Bayard Street, one block south of Canal.

That night, I was very lucky in that I got a parking spot for my 1970 Plymouth Barracuda on Canal Street right outside the Association. If I had not gotten that spot, I would have had to park along side the Manhattan Bridge, where they had 6 or 8 hour meters, the only ones longer than two hours in the area. These spots opened in the evening. So when I was going for a long stay, I always parked there. Anyhow, back to the story.

Professor Cheng, Tam Gibbs, and Ed Young were walking by, on their way to the Association. As they walked by, and we were getting out of the car, we came to Professor Cheng's attention. Since he looked our way, I walked over to him with my date, and introduced her. Professor said some Chinese words, laughed heartily, and walked away. I asked what had been said, and at first Tam said to us, "nothing important." My date lost interest, and left to go upstairs to get her seat in the anteroom so she could read during the class. I pressed Tam on what Professor meant, and he said quietly, so that she could not hear as she was walking away, the Professor said I would marry that girl.

On the one hand, Professor may have had a gift of foresight. On the other hand, if he did, he appeared to enjoy his knowledge of the difficulties that were coming my way over the course of an 18-year marriage.

Years later I asked her why she married me, since she did not like martial arts or movies. These were two of the three things I did the most, and the things she did with me, or watched with me, or attended with me, when we were dating. As soon as we were married, she stopped doing both. The best she could do was to say that she liked going out to eat with me.

One glance at my future, and eventual ex, wife, and Professor knew, without even needing to talk to her, she was not the right person for me. Later on, when things were bad, I wished that, back then, he had taken me aside and warned me. However, I thought that when I was suffering. In retrospect, I am not sure that I would have paid attention to his warning and taken his advice, as much as I respected Professor and his wisdom.

Ultimately he knew that everyone has to make their own mistakes in order to learn. And that by being challenged, we grow. Besides, two wonderful children came of that marriage.

Dues, the Value of Study with Professor Cheng

After I finished my second beginners' class, I was allowed to take more hours with Professor Cheng. As a beginner I had taken only form and the Friday night philosophy class lecture. It was $20.00 per contact hour with the Professor, so I paid $40.00 a month for the first two classes. As time went on, I paid over $120 a month in dues, which was a lot of money at the time. But I got to take form correction, push hands, sword form, dueling, calligraphy, and philosophy class with Professor, along with Chinese with Ed Young at an additional lesser monthly rate. As a cost comparison, my rent, starting at the time when I began my studies, was $75.00 per month. The rent went up to $88.00 a month by the time Professor passed. Transit fares were 20 cents a ride when I started class, and went up to 35 cents a ride during my years of studying with him. A hot dog was 15 cents, and a soda was a dime. And in a candy store, you could get a seltzer water with no syrup flavoring for 2 cents. You may have heard it called "For 2 Cents Plain." Dinner in Chinatown was 90 cents for beef and bok choy over rice.

I spent a lot of my salary on classes with Professor Cheng, but I very much wanted to learn. My take home pay was about $225 twice a month, so I paid about a quarter of my earnings to the school for instruction. I thought it was well worth every penny I spent to take classes with Professor Cheng.

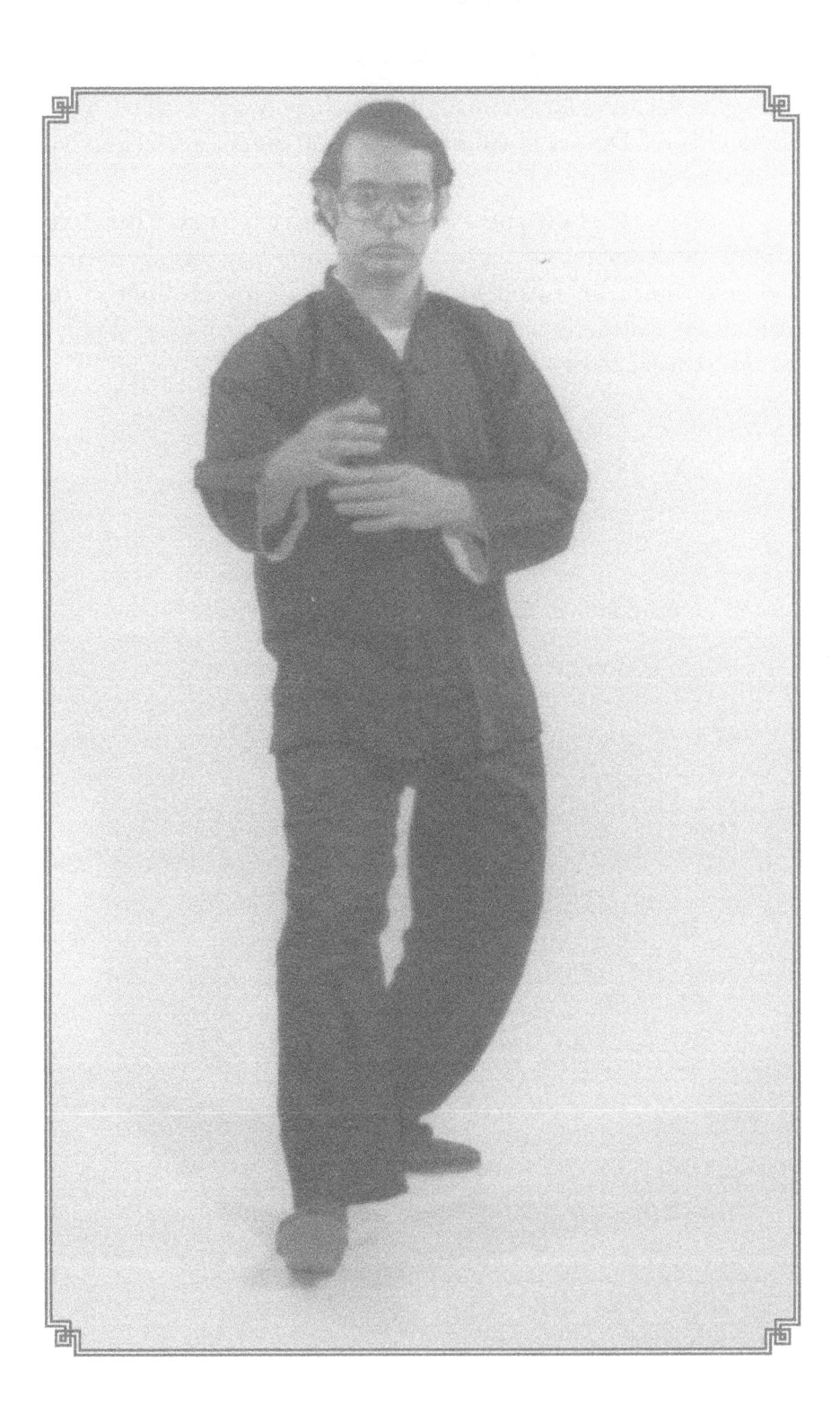

Chapter 5

Permissions and Media

I took notes

On Friday nights there were lecture classes. When I started T'ai Chi and heard about the classes from other students at the Association, I immediately wanted to attend, got permission, and paid for them.

Professor Cheng and Dr. Ren of Columbia University sat at a folding card table, and a portable blackboard was moved to just behind them. Professor taught and Dr. Ren translated. Professor Cheng wrote Chinese words on the board, and Dr. Ren translated, and sometimes Dr. Ren wrote English words on the board to explain the Chinese.

I sat in the back of the group class and took copious notes. I sat in the back because I was new, and I did not want to push ahead of those who were there already. Those people were senior to me, and had been taking the class before me. So as much as I really wanted to be in the front, I stayed in the back. The classes were on the teachings of Lao Tzu, and I was fascinated.

Audio permission

After that class ended another one started. This class was on Confucius, and I signed up for that as well. I was very eager to learn whatever Professor Cheng wanted to teach. I saw that a certain group of about 20 people were making audio recordings of the Professor at these lecture classes. So, when the Confucius class was announced, I asked for and received permission to make audiocassette tapes of the lectures and, additionally got permission to make tapes of the question and answer sessions that Professor would occasionally convene.

So I now had a reason to sit in the front. That reason was that Professor's lectures were long, longer than a ½ an hour side of an audiotape. I had to monitor my audiotape recorder. So, I sat in the first row to the left as I faced the table, and set up my microphone on the desk with all the others. While there must have been 20 microphones, all crowded together on that table, I came early and set mine up front and center. I used masking tape on the microphone's base, taping it to the table so it would not fall. Others making audiotapes were also sitting in the front, in the first three rows, at the other end of their microphone wires, so as to change their tapes.

Then Professor and Dr. Ren would come in and sit at the table. When Professor lectured, he spoke a few sentences at a time and then stopped so that Dr. Ren could translate. Sometimes Dr. Ren would ask questions in Chinese. Then, after a short conversation in Chinese, Dr. Ren would get the explanations, and then explain it to us. In addition to having the audiotape, I took extensive notes. Once in a while, when I was changing the audiotapes, Professor would pause so that I did not lose anything important. He rarely did that at all, but once in a while, he did it for me.

An eraser sat on the desk, for wiping the board clean. Once the eraser, which was on the left end of the desk, fell off the desk, and would have hit professor on one of his T'ai Chi slippers. He saw it fall and moved his foot, just a bit, and the eraser missed. I was amazed at his speed and timing. He moved his foot just out of the way, and also, he could not see through the desk, but he knew where the eraser would land.

I began to carry the tape player at all times, except when I forgot. You never knew when the Professor would just call a group around someone and start talking about what they were doing. He would then take questions, any questions, about T'ai Chi or anything else, from the assembled gathering. At the question and answer periods I may have been the only one taping, sometimes there may have been one or two others. I do not remember. But, as I have said, about 20 people had this permission. So, when Professor was set to give a formal lecture class, his table at the Association, and later the area in front of him at the Shr Jung, just bristled with microphones. I wonder where all the other tapes are today. I have my set.

A few years ago I won an argument because I had made those tapes. It was about the breathing in Professor's form. I knew how Professor Cheng wanted it done because I asked detailed questions about it (and, by the way, now provide that information in a download of the breathing available at PatienceTaiChi.com). The person I was trying to explain the breathing to had another idea. He was not having any of my knowledge, insisting that his theory was the correct way. At length, exasperated, I played my audiotape of me asking (and the translation into Chinese) and Professor answering my question (and the translation into English) about the breathing in that posture. Then, finally, it was a debate no longer.

Before I had this permission, and when I forgot my tape player, I was taking notes like crazy. Katy Cheng remembered at the "100th Anniversary of the Birth of Professor Cheng," (an event that I organized and hosted) that she recognized me because I was the one who was following her father around taking notes with pen or pencil and paper. I took notes on every scrap of paper I had, and I never had enough paper. First, I wrote right side up, in the lines of the paper, on both sides. Then, when the lines were filled, I wrote sideways in the margins, then upside down on the same side, between the lines of the notes I had previously written. I also wrote on business cards, and receipts and anything else I had that I could write on. I have those notes to this day, and, as you might imagine, they are hard to decipher, but still very precious.

Video

Permission to make film or video was another, more difficult matter. Only about six or seven people ever had that. Videotape was reel-to-reel at the time and very expensive, but I had a Super 8 camera and could make film of the Professor, if only I could get permission. So I asked for this permission as well, and I got more than I had asked for: I was permitted make film, and to take still pictures as well, with the Professor's approval.

I shot film for a while. From my beginner's perspective, dueling was the most advanced thing, so I got lots of film of dueling. Push hands came earlier in the permissions process, so I did not think it was as important as dueling. So I do not have much film of push hands. Boy do I regret that.

So, with full permission, why don't I have more material, you may ask? The reason is that I had some difficulty making film, even with the Professor's permission.

One day, when I was shooting film, someone who was there longer than I had been, and was therefore senior to me, stopped me from shooting the film. Knowing that you needed permission to film, he wanted to know what I thought I was doing. I told him I had permission to film. This got him angry. He walked right up to Professor Cheng and said, "How is it that he is filming and I can't? How is it that you did not give me permission and I have been here longer than him?" Professor told him through a translator that he gives permission or not for a reason. He gave me permission and not him, and it was not his business to question it. Professor then went on about his teaching, unbothered by the confrontation.

It traumatized me that a student would be so disrespectful and demanding of Professor Cheng. I was especially upset because the student was disrespectful because of me. I was upset that he was bothered because I was shooting film, and that is the reason I did not make more film. After that difficulty, I became shy about bringing my still or my film camera to the Association, as I did not want to make trouble for Professor Cheng. So I filmed little, and made that film as inconspicuously as possible. I also stopped taking photos until much later, in the Shr Jung, when I felt more confident that as a more senior person and eventually as a teacher there, I would not be the cause of trouble.

So, what was I to do? I wanted to take pictures and to make film so that I could look at them later on. I wanted to be able to learn from them later, and to remember the good times we had. As it happened, Stanley also had permission to make film. So I made an agreement with him, I would loan him my camera and supply the film to shoot Professor Cheng. No one would bother him as he shot the film, as no one was senior to him who did not have permission to film. This way, no one would confront Professor. I figured that this was a way that I could get the film I wanted, and not make any trouble for the Professor. In return, he agreed to make me copies of any film he shot of the Professor at the T'ai Chi Association with my camera and film. I then bought a case of Tri-X black and white film, 24 rolls, and gave it to Stanley. On my meager salary, and with what I was paying for classes, this was quite an investment. But Stanley started shooting the film, so I could get copies, and no more embarrassing situations for the Professor.

When the case of film was shot, I asked for my copies and my camera back. When I asked for my copies of the film, Stanley said, "Well, Bill, it's not such an easy matter to give copies to you." And then he fell back on his old saw, "It's complicated." This was his final response. He eventually returned the camera, broken, and some used and unused color cartridges. The used ones had fall foliage on them.

In the late '70s I had a friend who was a ju jitsu student in a school Stanley owned. He surprised me in front of a pizza place on

18th Avenue and 63rd Street one day. He ran up behind me and shouted. I turned, in a fighting stance, then saw it was a friend so we hugged and went to the back of the pizza place to eat slices of pizza and drink cokes. He told me that Stanley had shown a film of Professor Cheng at one of his dojos, upstairs, on 86th Street and 5th Avenue. That was my film.

Then in the late '80s or early '90s, Stanley did finally seem to be at the point of giving me a copy of the film. We were driving to a Chinese restaurant, taking our lunch break from Jou Tsung Hwa's Zhang San Feng Festival at the T'ai Chi Farm, and the conversation drifted on to Professor Cheng, and finally to the film he had shot with my camera. He asked me what I would do with the film if he made me a copy. When I said I would watch it, he seemed satisfied with my answer. But I did not leave well enough alone, foolish me. I added that I would give copies to my students. When I said that, alarm bells seemed to go off in his head. He asked me if I would really do that, as if it were a crime. He seemed confused by my desire to share it with my students. The upshot, he never got around to copying it for me, and I did not get that film in his lifetime.

When, in the fullness of time, he passed away, he left the film to Mario Napoli, or perhaps his wife just gave it to Mario, I do not know. But as I had said before, Stanley was a complicated man. The story has a happy ending. Mario Napoli, without knowing that the film was shot with my camera and film, or knowing of my deal with Stanley, gave me a copy of the film, which was in the form of a DVD. Thank you Mario.

The master tapes

While we are speaking about film and video, someone at the Association got hold of some really new technology for those days, a video recorder, and a Beta reel-to-reel videotape was made. By a twist of fate, I was absent, or out to eat, or something, almost every time they chose to shoot the videotape. An edited version of this video is available from the Cheng family, with interviews of many, including Maggie Newman, Ed Young and Ken Van Sickle. Ellen Cheng told me she had asked why I was not included in the interviews, and was told it was because I was not in the video. How that happened, I do not know. It was just not meant to be.

My friend Morgan Buchanan found some minor clips of me in the *Master Tapes* and forwarded information about them to me. It was not found in time, and at any rate, it was too minor an appearance. So I was not interviewed for the *Master Tapes*.

I was later interviewed for the movie, *The Professor, T'ai Chi's Journey West*, a film by Barry Strugatz. Not listed on the front cover is Kenneth Van Sickle, who was Professor Cheng's official photographer. He was also a driving force in the making of this movie.

THE MAGAZINE

I was not to be completely excluded from the "fame" of being in a public picture with Professor Cheng. In the summer of 1970, a reporter and cameraman from a Chinese magazine came by to do a pictorial and story on Professor. Ken Van Sickle took the pictures. I was included in a picture of my class of Professor's calligraphy students which was published in a 1971 issue of the magazine. I was so happy. Unfortunately for me, I had eaten cherry ices just before class. I looked like I was wearing lipstick. As I said, the picture was taken in the summer of 1970. The magazine came out in 1971, and I have a copy of it to this day. Mercifully the red has faded in the picture.

A CLASS PICTURE, THE FIRST

We were assembled to take a class picture in the Association. The photo would later appear in a yearbook kind of periodical that

Professor, or the Association, was putting out. I was new to the school and could not get a seat close to the front. Lenny Antonucci and I stood in the back. Then, suddenly, someone got up and I had the opportunity to sit in a back row. I took it. Lenny did not. So today you can see Lenny Antonucci standing in the back, but unless you know it's me, you can only guess where I am in that photo. Only my nose, eyes, eyeglasses, forehead and hair can be seen above the shoulders of the two people seated in front of me.

The second, third, and fourth class pictures

For the second class picture, I was prepared. I sat where my entire face could be seen. A third class picture was not published. I have gotten Kenneth Van Sickle's permission to publish it here. Hooray, you can see me. The fourth and last class picture was taken at the Shr Jung. I got a good place in that picture courtesy of Mort, who saved me a space, right next to him.

IN THE PRESENCE OF CHENG MAN-CH'ING

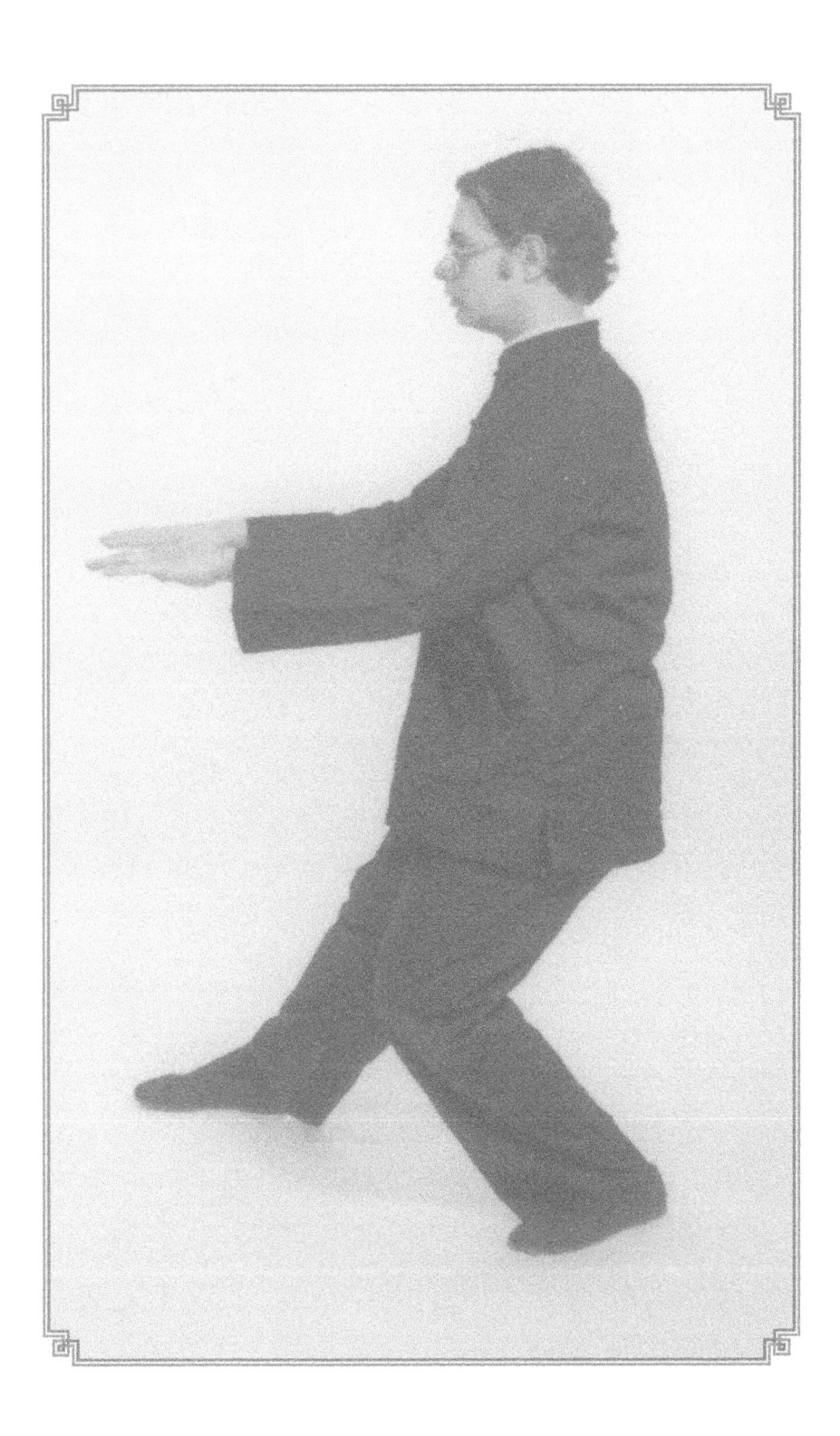

Chapter 6

More Stories from the Association

Driving Professor to the school, kung fu in the car

I was lucky in this. My class on was a weekday, early evening, but I always went to the school on Sundays as well, to watch, to hang out, and to soak up what I could of information, atmosphere, and culture. I was not there very long when they asked for a volunteer to pick up Professor at his apartment and drive him to the T'ai Chi Association at 211 Canal Street on Sunday in the late mornings. Though I lived in the southern end of Brooklyn and picking him up meant going to the northern end of Manhattan, I immediately volunteered. I found it to be an honor and a privilege to be allowed to drive him. I think he lived, if memory serves, on Riverside Drive and West 104th Street. Though I never saw it, I was told he had a westerly-facing apartment on a high floor. The view was of the Hudson River, with spectacular sunsets. I waited with the car on the street for Professor, and whoever was with him.

He would always be accompanied by Ed or Tam, sometimes both. Occasionally there would be another. They came out of his building and got into my car, Professor would sit in the back with the students, and if necessary, a student would sit next to me in the passenger seat. They would typically be talking animatedly in Chinese while I drove them down town to the T'ai Chi Association in Chinatown.

Driving the Professor on Sundays gave me additional contact with him, for which I was very happy. However, it led to the following misapprehension and intense personal embarrassment: Once, as I was driving downtown, I heard my name mentioned. In the same sentence or phrase as my name were the words kung fu and a flurry of words I did not understand, all in Chinese.

Naturally, I got excited. Was he preparing to tell me a secret of kung fu? Was that to be my reward for driving him? Did I know something about kung fu that he was praising? So I quickly and impolitely interrupted and asked.

I was told that he had said that I should use more discipline in my driving. What about the words kung fu that I had heard, I eagerly wondered out loud. The answer was: it means discipline, as when American martial artists say, "He studies the art," and we know they are referring to a martial art, when Chinese refer to "discipline", they are referring sometimes to a specific discipline—martial art. However, in this case Professor was not. He was referring to the lack of self-discipline in my driving. I was hitting far too many potholes as I drove. My chest fell, my ego deflated.

So I slowed down, drove carefully, and did not hit too many more potholes thereafter. I was duly chastened.

It was the first time, but not the last time that I embarrassed myself in front of the Professor.

Professor would just call a talk

At the Association and at the Shr Jung after, Professor would sometimes just call a talk, and we would gather around and listen. Most of the time classes stopped when Professor was talking. We just wanted to hear what he had to say. Here are several of those stories as I remember them.

He told us that once, during WW2, he was sitting on his porch and a Chinese freedom fighter ran past, and went to the left. A little later a Japanese patrol came by, on the trail of the freedom fighter. The officer asked Professor which way the man had run. Without any hesitation, the Professor said the man had run by his house and turned to the right. As a result, the officer leading the patrol pursued the man in that direction.

Professor used this as a lesson in how to be honest: You should not get someone killed for the sake of your honesty, so that you can, out of a sense of vanity, tell people that you never told a lie. You have to judge your words. He said he never lost any sleep over this incident, and we should not either, in the same kind of situation as this. We need to see honesty in this light.

The moral of the story is not to obsess over the "truth", but do no harm with your words. Don't tell the truth, or a lie, to get someone harmed. Don't tell the truth for no good reason, except your love of the truth. He said we should not get all caught up with the truth, but use words so they do no harm. He said that is the truth, the higher truth.

I believe he spent much of the war with Chiang Kai-shek in Chungking, training troops, so I do not know if this ever happened. (Not that it is my place to know.) It may have happened, or maybe he was just telling us this story to illustrate his point. But if it did happen, he never regretted it and considered himself to be an honest man.

He told of how he escaped from the Communists, to Taiwan, with just 10 trunks, and lost his favorite feather fan as he fled. But he had his life, and he never regretted the loss of things. Perhaps a lesson in materialism.

He told us of one of his students in Taiwan. He said that the student learned "it" in six months. Professor used that story to let us know that while some can learn "it" fast, the rest of us need to learn "it" slowly. However, he never explained exactly what "it" was, though I assumed that "it" was what he was trying to teach us all the time: to relax.

He told us of another student in Taiwan. This student was an old man, but could have rifle barrels shoved into his gut, or his kidneys, with no ill effect. Professor said the man sometimes needed help to stand up, but once up, and braced against a wall, or a tree, no one could hurt him by punching him, or poking him with a rifle barrel.

Looking back, I wonder if we were told what "it" was, and "it" was just not translated. Katy Cheng has said Professor was often not well translated, as he spoke in a literary form and the translators often had to do double duty, translate what he said into every day Chinese and then, to translate that into English.

Language Class

Ed Young taught Chinese, but Professor was there and made a comment from time to time. One of the word groups we learned, and had explained to us, were the words for T'ai Chi Ch'uan: supreme ultimate fist or boxing. A double character word we later learned, was wife: t'ai t'ai. I thought, since t'ai means supreme, and t'ai t'ai is wife, and it was written as t'ai twice (so it was not me misunderstanding tones), being married was a special blessing in traditional Chinese culture. I asked about it. I was right. :-)

Lest you think I was getting really good at this: Mah is question (interrogative). The traditional way to ask if you are well, or how are you, or 'how you doin?" to put it in a neighborhood New York vernacular is "ni how mah" (you well<interrogative>). But this word mah, can, with a different tone, mean horse. The two mahs are even written almost the same. Add a mouth symbol to the word for question and you have a horse. I remembered it by thinking of the old American saying, still current at that time, "Do not look a gift horse in the mouth."

Anyhow, I often greeted Chinese friends, with "You good horse." It was embarrassing, so I eventually used a vernacular way of asking: "how bu how," which means literally, "well no (not) well", and comes to the same thing in Chinese. And so, I stopped calling classmates good horses.

Marina Cheng teaches me

I made no secret of the fact that I was an English teacher in high school, as well as a martial artist. Marina, one of Professor's daughters, asked me to help her with her English. She offered to pay me, but I asked that she teach me something in exchange. When she mentioned the things she could teach me something about, I selected Five Element theory. We taught each other in the anteroom of the Association. It ended, and I do not remember why. I l liked Marina, she was sweet, and patient with me. I was so eager to share what I knew, and learn, from her. She passed away way too soon.

Calligraphy class, or tic-tac-toe

I signed up for calligraphy class with Professor. I thought I would be writing words with a brush. Not so fast. First we learned how to make ink. We put a few drops of water into our ink-making ceramic thingy. Then we took an ink stick and started rubbing it in circles, on the thingy, until the bottom of the stick dissolved into ink. When the liquid turned black we were not finished. The ink had to be of the appropriate thickness, or consistency.

When we got good enough at that, or Professor realized we were not going to get any better, Professor had us take a page of the New York Times (any full-sized section), and put it in front of us. Then he had us draw horizontal lines across the page. We held our left hands on the page, palm open and down, and with the brush in our right hands, moved our tan t'iens in a small move from left to right. As we did this, we drew our right hands all the way across the page. Our hands were pulled by our tan t'iens. That way the lines were straight and even. He also wanted us to end the lines without trailing off, but to go back over the end of the line and make it even as well. He asked us to keep the pages. I had no idea why.

Then, when we had done that for a few weeks, he had us get the papers we had saved, the sheets with the horizontal lines, and begin to draw vertical lines. Same idea, we drew our tan t'iens down to pull our brush hands down. When we had done all the pages, and had a grid of squares, he had us draw circles within the squares. It kind of tickled, moving my tan t'ien in such a small circle. Then we drew X's over the circles. I regret that I got no farther than that in this class. It came to an end, I do not remember why. Maggie Newman was a senior classmate in this class.

On Posture and Form

Professor Cheng had a very clear idea of what he wanted in a posture and in the form at any given time. I say at any given time because in his early pictures, he looks a lot more martial than he did later. Just my opinion, but I think that as he improved over the decades, he became softer and it showed in his form. He was precise because the form is Chinese Yoga for health as well as martial arts, to save our lives, and in either, a mistake of an inch can negate any benefit. It must be done with exactitude.

But a problem in our T'ai Chi is people who learn it from people who learned it from people who learned. it. I could go on, but you get the picture. What goes in is sometimes not the same as what comes out. Sometimes things seem to get lost, and other things to appear in the students of teachers in this category. If they are open to being helped, it is our duty to help them.

I might add here that really good form is rare, and two of the best forms that I have seen are done by Maggie Newman, and by Joanne Chang, a student of Ben Lo.

It's funny, but at the T'ai Chi Gala, one of my fellow presenters said that his form was not as good as mine, and then demonstrated. I told him I am not the T'ai Chi police because I did not want to be an intimidating presence, especially to my friends. Perhaps

I would have done him a better service by offering to correct, rather than accepting what he was doing. My motivation was that I always want to be a friendly, approachable person, especially to people who I like.

Knowing the variations became very important as I judge Cheng Man-Ch'ing division T'ai Chi forms at tournaments. Knowing the teacher often explains the variation, and there are more methods than I have noted above. Professor had students in east Asia, Malaysia, and Indonesia, who also have students who settled here, in the USA and Canada. They have their methods. They all deserve a fair shake at tournaments.

Professor and his video

Professor Cheng gave us much better and more detailed correction than you could ever see in any of his videos. I do not know if he was just uninterested in having his knowledge out on video, or he was keeping the good stuff for those of us who learned in person. I have wondered about this and discussed it with a number of people. My final opinion: he did not want you to be able to learn from a video. He wanted you to study, with him or with a student, to really learn what he wanted to teach.

For example, in films he never sank deeply into squatting single whip (snake creeps up, or down, name it as you will), and so a couple of people who use the video as a bible of what is right and wrong took issue with me on this posture. However, while I could not convince them of what I was taught, I was able to show them the still photo taken for the Taiwanese consulate's piece on Chinese Martial Arts. They saw him taking a low position and stopped debating with me about the posture. In any case, I know what I was taught, and do it, and teach it, regardless of criticism, especially from people who learned Cheng Man Ch'ing's T'ai Chi from a book or one of Professor's videos. I was there, and learned Cheng Man-Ch'ing's T'ai Chi from Cheng Man-Ch'ing as he wanted it to be. Enough said.

On breath

I learned the breathing. I do not like to blow my own horn, but I may be one of the very few people who got it from Professor because I thought it was important and asked. He told everyone to inhale on yang moves, and exhale on yin moves, but he never explained his breathing publicly beyond that, that I am aware of. He also never explained, in my hearing, what a yin move was and what a yang move was. I do think most people understood what he meant by that. This explanation still left a lot to the imagination. Not having much imagination, I asked. First, I asked questions about the breathing in the parts of the form I did not understand. Eventually I asked about the breathing in the parts I thought I did understand as well, just to be sure, and there were a couple of surprises. So much for what I thought I knew. As mentioned earlier, at Patience T'ai Chi (PatienceTaiChi.com) we have a downloadable recording of the breathing instruction, the only instructional download extant on breathing in the Professor Cheng's form that I am aware of.

According to Professor Cheng, the breathing is precise and the breathing is important. He just could not get people to become interested in the breathing. They were only interested in the "secrets," and breathing, secret or not, was not what they were interested in. So they reserved their interests to learning the "secrets" of form, push hands, sword form, dueling, and fighting. He was fond of saying that there are no secrets. There was so much information that he had, and would share for the asking. All you had to do was ask. I recognized that and asked.

On training the legs

Many people talk about standing postures and some ask if Professor taught us to stand. I have to say, "No.... but..."

Without specifically teaching standing postures, Professor would kill us with his technique of correcting a large class: There were sometimes up to 100 people in each of his classes at the Shr Jung, and he corrected slowly, one at a time. By the time he was finished correcting, you were exhausted. It was up to you how deep you stood, and many a stance got deeper just before the Professor arrived at someone's spot.

I always took deep stances, but watched out for him whenever I hit my fatigue level. If he had his back turned, I stood up for a few seconds and released my legs from the pressure they were under in those stances. I always tried not to be seen out of posture. However when I did this, he seemed to know, almost psychically. He would turn and look, as I was dropping back down, refreshed a bit, till the next time. It was obvious that he knew what I and some others, were doing. Perhaps he was amused by it, but he never reprimanded us.

My legs were strong when I studied T'ai Chi. When I arrived at the Shr Jung for advanced form correction class, I climbed the four or five flights effortlessly (we were on the top floor of 87 Bowery). Yet, after a class with the Professor, I had to hold the banister going down the stairs, my legs were so fatigued and rubbery. I just about fell down those stairs, as my legs could not hold me up on the way out, in spite of the fact that I had run cross country for 2½ years in high school, and then did ju jitsu, sport judo with its ouchi komi exercises, and tai sabaki, throw for throw, randori and karate with its horse stances, and deep stance punching and kicking for years after that. Those practices had exhausted my legs, and as I got used to them, they made them stronger. In the T'ai Chi advanced correction, I started strengthening them all over again.

CH'I AND ME

The first time I felt ch'i was a monumental event for me. It was this nice tingle in the fingers. But when I told anyone, my nervousness about it made the feeling go away for days. When I relaxed enough, I could feel it again. Often, when it returned, it would come back at the most unusual of times. I remember one time it came back as I was about to drive through Prospect Park from the Flatbush Avenue side on a bright warm sunny summer day.

Later, in conversation, through a translator of course, during a medical consultation—which was when I often had conversations with him—Professor told me to do the raise hands back and down for an hour a day. No explanation, just do it. I did it. After a while I felt ch'i, uninterrupted ch'i, and no amount of talking about it could make it go away. I did the extra hour of practice of the ch'i exercise for about six months. This is the reason that to this day, I call the raise hands back and down, the "ch'i exercise."

I hope the name catches on. Several other things that I have said have become part of the terminology of explanations of T'ai Chi. For example, I used the phrase: T'ai Chi is a slow motion moving meditative exercise, a Chinese yoga. Now it is common to hear it called both of those things: moving meditation and Chinese yoga.

I should point out that he never told me to stop doing the raise hands back and down, or to do it for only six months. I stopped myself when I thought I had gotten enough from the practice. Also, the ch'i exercise did not take the place of any other exercise. It was additional practice, in my already quite busy day. That was why I stopped. Having gotten a good benefit, I felt I could better use the time for other things.

Banquets

I attended three of them. The first one was in the back room of a restaurant. I'm not sure where the restaurant was, maybe on Canal street. You entered the restaurant and walked to the back of the dining area, and then through the kitchen. There was another dining area behind the kitchen. I wondered if the back room behind the kitchen was a leftover from Prohibition.

The dishes at that banquet were the basic (like chicken and peas, or chicken and celery), and the exotic, which I would never eat. I do not remember what the menu was beyond that I ate the former, and not any of the latter.

About the second banquet, I do not remember the place or the menu. What I remember about it was that it was in a fluorescent lit, private room. A major feature of this banquet was the presence of a special guest: Swami Bua. He and Professor Cheng seemed to know and respect each other. They ate and drank together, communicated somehow, and had a good time. At that banquet scotch was served and the Professor drank a lot of it, but was not the least bit drunk.

It is interesting to note Swami Bua's indirect but definite influence on my life. When I next saw the Swami, the Professor had passed on and I was at a Festival of Yoga and Esoteric Science that Dr. Douglas Baker and Mr. Tony Fisichella were taking around the world. I went to see it in Long Island, NY. I went because Swami Bua was teaching there. His presence told me that the event was probably on the level, as, at that time, I knew no one else who was speaking or demonstrating.

Swami Bua also affected Mario Napoli, the student I mentioned before of Stan Israel's maturity. I do not know how he found the Swami, but he studied with him.

At that time, on Long Island, I saw some of the skill of Swami Bua. Though he was old, he was able to sit in a full lotus on a table at the front of the lecture room, and he appeared comfortable. On the other hand, at lecture classes at the Shr Jung, I occasionally sat in a full lotus for a few minutes, because I saw Professor Cheng sitting very comfortably in one. Then I changed to a half lotus and if the class was long, I pretended to have to go to the bathroom, so that I could stretch my legs.

The second thing that I remember that the Swami did was to take a handkerchief and stick it up one nostril and pull it down the other. I was amazed. Though my nose may be stuffed, I have never wanted it cleared enough to do that to it. Swami demonstrated many other skills that day.

The third banquet was memorable to me because it was held in a modern restaurant. There were fish tanks of exotic fish (not fish to eat, but fish to look at). I do, however, remember one of the exotic dishes: duck fat. When I asked someone about that, I was told that the Chinese peasant did not get much fat in their diet and it was special when they could. I tried it. Even with all the hot dog fat I was eating, it was still too much for me.

Professor stands for tolerance

I was not going to use this story in the book, but since Ken Van Sickle has me talking about it on camera, and then put it into the movie, *The Professor, T'ai Chi's Journey West*, here it is, the whole story.

When Professor was visiting in Taiwan, the Association closed us out of the school. They could not do this openly to Professor's face, apparently, but in his absence they told us to go. They had not been happy that an important part of Chinese culture was being shown to non–Chinese. When questioned about this, they said they accepted white people, grudgingly and black people as well, without too much of a fuss. But, make no mistake, they were not happy about it. Remember earlier, when I told the story of when I showed up looking for Professor, I was basically told to go away until Professor intervened.

That was not the problem that got us put out. It was a student of Japanese extraction that Professor had accepted. For that student, they put us all out and kept us out. It was too close to WW2, and to the rape of Nanking and other Japanese atrocities that had been done to the Chinese people during the war. Our Japanese student was not a part of that, in fact our student was Nisei, or second generation American, a citizen. She is a very gentle, peaceful human being as well. But the board of the T'ai Chi Association did not feel that way about it. She was just a Japanese to them. We all gathered outside the Association on Canal Street, milling about and wondering what to do. One of the senior students, perhaps it was Ed Young, called Professor in Taiwan and asked what we should do. Professor told him that we should start another school and he would come back to us. So, you may ask, was our Japanese student that important to Professor, or was it the principle that prejudice is wrong? My guess is both. To this day that student teaches, living up to the promise Professor may have seen.

Crosby Street

When we were told to form a school and Professor would come back to us upon his return to New York City, it was not as easy as that. The senior students had to a rent space for us to use immediately, and also save to rent a new space for us to move to. They did this while also accumulating the money that would be needed to fix the new place up, as it would be Professor's New York headquarters. In answer to the immediate problem, they rented temporary space on Crosby Street. Shortly after they rented the space to which we would move the school to. After the summer, when the work was done, the senior students moved us into what would be called, "The Shr Jung" on the top floor of 87 Bowery.

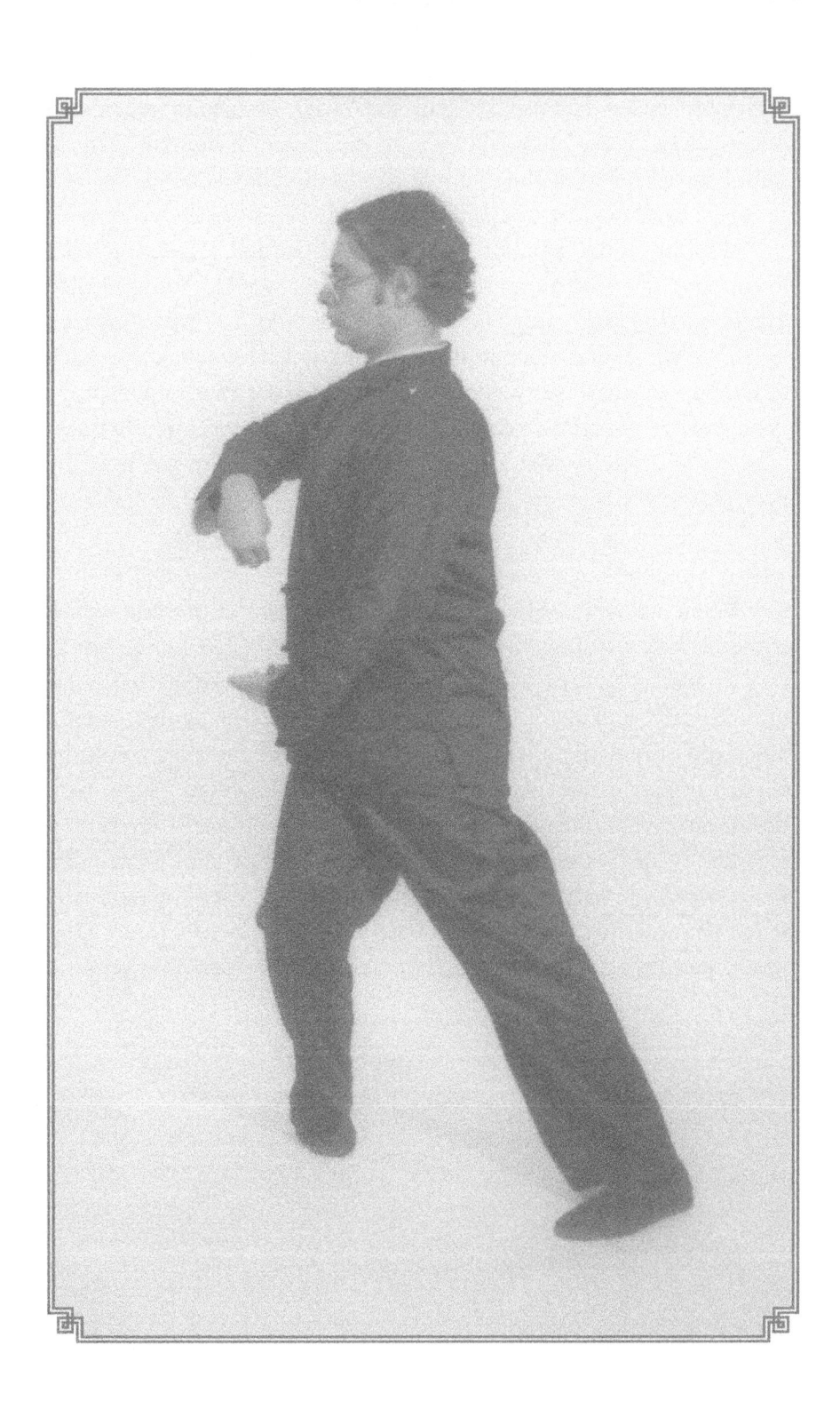

Chapter 7

Shr Jung

The Association, at 211 Canal Street, in Manhattan, was a suite of two rooms. One was the front room, where Professor had a desk, in front of which was a table and wooden chairs. This was where calligraphy was taught. If nothing was going on, you could sit there, eat lunch, read, or just hang out. At the foot of the table was a comfortable chair with a green plastic seat and back. The second room was the main room, large and rectangular. A mirror was on the wall that separated it from the office, and there was a wall with south facing windows onto Canal Street. There were three lines of chairs for spectators along the window wall. Push hands was played against the opposite wall from the office. The fourth wall had an air conditioner in the window, just short of it were the bathrooms. In front of the bathrooms there was a sword rack.

The Shr Jung on the other hand, was one long floor through loft from east to west. There were windows onto the Bowery, the west side of the Shr Jung. On the north side there was a brick wall all the way down to the back, where the sink was on the north wall, just short of the east wall. Mirrors were on that north wall, from about seventy feet in. The front was a push hands area.

On the south side, there was a large walk-in storage closet constructed of wood. Past that was Professor's desk, and the display cabinet, then there were bathrooms and the entrance from the top of the stairs. Further into the building was the area where we sat for Professor's lectures. When there was no class opposite, in front of the mirrors, it was another push hands area. At the back (east wall) there was a sink and a table, where calligraphy was practiced and tea could be had.

It was near the Bowery windows that I taught my beginners class on Sunday. Ed Young taught an advanced or correction class in front of the mirrors.

When the place was first rented, it needed renovations

Harold Naiderman did the electrical work. He ran the electrical lines and put in the lights. I wanted to be of help in the renovation but had no special skills and so I started to assist Harold. I helped him by holding wire and fetching things for him, and that was how we became friends that hot and sweaty summer and fall.

Jon Gaines also worked on the renovation. He did carpentry. Herman Kauz did a lot of work as well, though I do not remember what he did, as I did not help him do it. I often saw him there, busily doing stuff. Several others wandered in and out, taking care of things at our new home. But most of the students were not available to help.

Professor's students were mainly of three types, hippies, martial artists, and none of the above. We martial artists called them civilians. The hippies typically lived in the East Village and came to Professor for spiritual knowledge, as well as T'ai Chi. The martial artists came for fighting, or because of Professor's martial skill. I was one of those, though I also came for the medicine, spiritual knowledge and whatever else Professor wanted to teach. As for the others, who knows what they came for? But one thing you could be sure of, when Professor was away, so were most of them. There were those that felt that, since they paid their dues, they did not have to help with anything. So it was only those of us who felt that it was our T'ai Chi duty to fix up our T'ai Chi home and be of service to Professor who stepped up and took care of whatever needed to be done. When Professor was due back, most of the others returned, some even before he arrived.

Herman Kauz stands up for the school

When work on the new school at 87 Bowery was finished and we had begun starting classes at the Shr Jung, and after word went out that the Professor was coming back (but before he actually came back and joined us, and not the Association), those students who had left when he left, as well as those who left when we moved to our temporary location on Crosby Street, started to filter back in.

When we had a crowd of them, there was a general meeting of all students. During the meeting, some of the students asked, rebelliously, why did they have to follow the senior students when doing the form in class at the school. They had the idea that they could do form as well as anyone, including their seniors. They thought they should take turns leading. There was general agreement with this sentiment among those gathered. No one wanted to stand up to the students. Though senior students were present, they did not speak up.

Herman, who was passing by the meeting while doing some final work on the Shr Jung, stepped into the gap. He put it to them bluntly: "You do the form in the school by following us because we know the form better than you do. You follow your betters and learn from us. This school is not a democracy, but a learning experience, for those of you who wish to learn." He personally put down the potential rebellion. Then he left the meeting and continued on with whatever work he was doing, preparing the Shr Jung for Professor's return. He kept the school together, under its leadership, and single handedly prevented it from breaking into factions. Shortly after that Herman left the school. I do not know why.

Professor's Return

We were very happy when Professor came back to us and began to teach and give medicine again. As a byproduct, classes grew tremendously when he was home with us. One reason that Professor's correction class was very hard at the Shr Jung was because there were so many students in it. We would stay in postures for twenty to thirty minutes, while Professor corrected. Great for the legs, in retrospect.

Medicine

Early on in my studies, I went to Professor for oriental diagnosis and herbal medicine. At the Association, when I was driving him to the school, he saw me for medicine at no charge. I did not appreciate what an honor that was, until I went for medicine at the Shr Jung when I was not driving him. At the Shr Jung he charged me $15 dollars a session, I think that was his going rate.

When I joined the Association, in spite of my busy schedule (or perhaps because of it), my health was weak and I ran high fevers and had illnesses. At that time, while I was studying T'ai Chi, I was going to work as a New York City high school teacher, going to graduate school, and teaching ju jitsu, judo, and karate. In addition, I had allergies. So I was very fortunate that I got to see him for herbal medicine. He always knew what to prescribe, and he took good care of me.

A prescription consisted of three packages. You opened one and put it in a pot. You then added three cups of water and boiled it down to one cup. This took about 45 minutes. Then you drank it. For your next dose, you again added three cups and boiled it down to one, and it took about an hour the second time. And then you drank that.

The first time I took the medicine, which tasted pretty much like what it looked like, forest floor, I was at my Grandmother's house. It went down, and my stomach lurched. The medicine turned around and tried to come back up. I closed my mouth and my throat and gagged to keep it down. I was successful, just barely.

The filled prescription came with six little packages of white (yellow) raisins to take, one package after each dose of medicine. It was not enough. Ice cream would not have been enough. But the medicine worked and I felt better after taking it, so I drank it.

He took my pulses in the Chinese way, 3 in each wrist, with three pressures for each pulse. He could see not only what was wrong with me, but how it got that way, as well as what my future held. On one occasion he told me I had developed my allergies because I had a sickness when I was about five. In fact, I was very sick when I was five and my Mom kept me home with a low-grade fever. After a couple of months of that, she just sent me back to school, because I never got any better at home. Whatever I had went undiagnosed and, according to Professor, eventually became my allergies.

One time, at the Association, when I went to him for medicine, he asked me about my diet. I told him that I ate about 20 pounds of meat a week, mostly hot dogs, except when I could afford the occasional hamburger. He then told me about his diet and that I should work to improve my diet. As a result, he motivated me to start to change my diet.

For me, dinner was, and still is, my big meal, though it gets competition from breakfast these days. I made my first attempt, or baby step, on the way to eating well at that time. I have never stopped working on improving my diet. I was not a grain or a vegetable eater. The first step in my changing diet was dinner. I started eating beef on rice at Sum Hey Rice shop in Chinatown. It cost 90 cents. I could have eaten my fill of three hot dogs for 45 cents. So I was investing in myself. I did not like rice at first, I had to get used to it. Then I graduated to beef, bok choy and mixed vegetables with tofu on rice, for $1.25. Fresh Chinese green vegetables came easier to me than the rice did. It was the American staples, like canned peas and carrots and string beans I did not like. I do not like canned veggies to this day.

I was not that good at what I ate for years and am still improving. There were a lot of tasty diversions in Chinatown that never made it to my local Chinese restaurant. Most notably among them was cha shu bao. It was a baked bread roll, with pork and a sweet sauce inside. Not particularly good for health, (especially if you did not know about the paper on the bottom and ate it) but wonderful to the taste buds.

For information about Professor's diet, see page 80.

One time at the Shr Jung, while taking my pulses, Professor asked me what I was doing in my life. I answered that I did not know. He also asked about women, and I answered that I did not have much luck. He then asked about what I was reading and I told him. I knew that I had had a wonderful opportunity to impress him, but that I had answered badly. I think he knew by this time that I was going to be a teacher of his form, and I think that he asked more because he wanted to know if I knew it. Perhaps he thought he could elicit the information from me. It was then that he invited me to always ask any questions that I wanted to ask. I had already been asking a lot of questions, more than Tam and Ed were comfortable with, this was an invitation to ask even more. Boy, did I ever use that privilege.

Another time, at a medical consultation, he asked me how I felt when he was jolting me with electric "ch'i" current out of his hands as he took my "Chinese pulses." I told him it felt like I was plugged into an electric socket. He smiled. He was healing me energetically, even as he listened for my imbalances so he could prescribe herbs.

Others Received Medicine as Well

I do not want to give the impression that I was the only one getting medicine or that it was a privilege. Professor would do as many as 20 medical sessions a day, both at the Association and later, at the Shr Jung. He would probably have done more but was limited by Ed and Tam. They wanted to protect Professor and not let him get too tired. Most got prescriptions. Some got Professor's ch'i. I got both.

One time a student had a broken leg. I do not remember all the details of the break. The student had X-ray pictures taken and a caste was put on before he saw Professor. Professor put his hands on the student's leg and sent ch'i there, and the student felt a lot better. Feeling better, the student went back for more X–rays, and the doctor was astounded. The student said his doctor said that three months of healing had happened that day between the first and second X–rays.

I once brought a friend to see the Professor for medicine. Tam did not like that at all, wasting Professor's time and energy on a non-student, but Professor did not seem to mind. He told my friend that he had a venereal disease. My friend had not tested as such in western medicine, and did not think he had a venereal disease. But he took the herbs that Professor prescribed, and was indeed feeling better after.

I once asked the apothecary that filled Professor's prescriptions if he could understand Professor's herbal medicine. After all, he filled the prescriptions. I could not understand how the forest floor he was preparing for me to boil and drink: roots, mud, leaves, small berry-looking things, twigs, moss and seeds etc. became medicine. The Chinese pharmacist at the herbal store answered a question I had not thought to ask, instead of the one I had asked. He answered that though he was a doctor of Chinese medicine himself, and filled the prescriptions Professor wrote, he had no clue as to how they worked. Professor, he said, was a doctor of Traditional Chinese Medicine like he was. But he had no idea how the herbs Professor gave me, when combined as he was combining them, had any beneficial effect. It was beyond his understanding of his craft. And so I got more of an answer than I had asked for. I just wanted to know how herbs worked, as at the time, for me, medicine came from a pharmacy, a drug company. This man, who also wrote prescriptions out of the same stuff as Professor, was praising him to the sky. But then, Professor's skill was just that high.

Professor Cheng typically gave me a prescription for three and on rare occasions, 6 days of medicine to fix whatever ailed me. It worked, unfailingly. Professor's medicine, along with the T'ai Chi, left me feeling that I was in the best health of my life.

However, when Professor was leaving for Taiwan that last time he wrote me a renewable scrip. I had never had a renewable script before. It lowers my temperature by half a degree if I have a fever, and if my temperature is normal, it does nothing.

Professor's rubbing medicine

Professor Cheng also had his own dit da jou, or rubbing medicine. You could drink it, and Tam did. If drunk, I was told it had a toning effect on the system. Tam said it raised his ch'i. I never tried it, I did not have enough to use it that way. It was miraculous stuff. When he brought it to the Shr Jung, it was a light brown powder, which looked a lot like tanic acid, a staple of my chemistry set when I was a youngster. He would mix it with scotch (Johnny Walker Black Label) and it would heal what hurt you, even if you rubbed it on the location of an old and persistent pain. Even then, the pain would subside.

This quality of it being drinkable, and our faith in it, is thought to have played a part in the death of senior student Tam Gibbs. Tam had a bad stomach ache and decided to self-treat by drinking the dit ta jou. It was a tragically wrong thing to do. His stomach problem was appendicitis, and he died of it.

I was given a four-ounce bottle of the stuff, and it worked on a scar I had inflicted on myself when I was a teen, maybe 10 years earlier, when I became a "blood brother" at a sleep away camp.

I cut my hand, in the meat, under my thumb, and it had been scarred and sore ever after. One drop and the decade or so of persistent pain was gone. It was that good, and so I also used it on myself and my ju jitsu and karate students' pains whenever we bruised ourselves and the bruise/and or the pain would not go away after a reasonable time. The dit da jou lasted throughout the late '70s and into early '80s. Finally when I began to run out, I diluted it with more scotch. After a couple of dilutions it lost its strength.

I wish I had some of that stuff today. Now, I am lucky enough to have access to Dale Dugas' dit da jou and it is better than anything else I have found since I ran out of Professor's. But is not anywhere near as good as Professor's dit da jou.

A friend of a friend knows someone who has several bottles of Professor's dit da jou, but considers it a valued shrine or collector's item and will not use it or sell a bottle, even for hundreds of dollars. I will say right here and now I will pay him. If he agrees, I will have it analyzed and, if possible, have more made.

Otherwise, the secret died with Professor Cheng.

Medicine after Professor

After Professor passed, I had no easy source of Traditional Chinese Medical prescriptions. Eventually I mentioned this to the second apothecary, to whom Professor had sent us to fill the prescriptions he wrote. He agreed to take my pulses the Chinese way and prescribe for me. I told him how Professor Cheng knew all about me and my life's illness from the pulses. He said that he could barely tell how I was doing now from the pulses. He said that he filled Professors prescriptions but did not know how they worked. He had no idea of Professor's understanding except that it was way beyond his own. And he said that he thought he, himself, was a good practitioner. This was a second dose of high praise for Professor's medical knowledge.

I brought him three of my friends for herbal medicine. He

agreed to see them because of me, though he was nervous about it because he was afraid of being accused of practicing medicine without a license. He saw them repeatedly and eventually gave them a year's worth of medicine. But he did not have the same kind of effect that Professor had in three days. So high was Professor's understanding. And so I add my praise for Professor's medicine.

After that, I brought another friend to the apothecary, but the shop had changed, and where there were boxes of herbs, there was toothpaste and mouthwash. The man would not even speak English to me. He pretended that he did not speak English. I wonder if prescribing for an American had brought difficulty to him for his willingness to help. My friend Alex was the only one who felt better after a year.

Professor's diet

Professor told us of his diet, though I never saw him eat, except at banquets. He said he ate congee, which is rice boiled until it becomes a loose soup, for breakfast at 6:00 AM. He ate green vegetables and rice with peanuts at noon and congee again at 6:00 PM. He said that you should eat the big meal in the middle of the day. He added that he drank some blackberry brandy on cold mornings to get his ch'i flowing.

However, he ate and drank whatever was put in front of him at banquets and social events, and he probably enjoyed the variety, too.

While he would abstain in his personal life, at a banquet, he would drink anyone under the table. He could drink Scotch whiskey almost endlessly, and not be drunk. This makes me wonder if he had any alcohol drinking skill beyond a natural talent.

This led some people to misunderstand what they saw at banquets. They believed that he had a drinking problem.

From where I sit, he did not. In his personal life he was the most ascetic person that I ever met.

On Questions for Professor

Professor had encouraged me to ask as many questions as I wanted to. After he did that, I knew I could always go back again and ask again if I was not sure. The barrier between me and learning fell. I did not have to wait for a special event, or an auspicious time, to ask a question, and I got a lot of valuable information just by asking. For example, I asked about the breathing in the form. I wanted to know all the inhales and all the exhales of the form. The general information Professor provided to the class, was just not enough for me.

I am sure that I made even more of a pest of myself. Pretty soon Tam asked me to go away and would not ask my questions. Then Ed got tired of me asking. Tam and Ed said I was tiring Professor out and hogging his time, but Professor always seemed happy that I asked, and he was patient with me.

What to do? At the Shr Jung, I asked Morty's wife, Ling Raphael, to translate my questions, and she always did whenever Tam and Ed would not. Professor continued patiently and happily to answer. He never thought I was a pest. Stupid maybe, but not a pest. In fact, on the occasion of the Friday night of the weekend Celebration of the 100th Anniversary of the Birth of Professor Cheng Man–Ch'ing, when we were sharing our memories of Professor Cheng and our time studying with him, Katy Cheng, one of Professor's daughters, remembered me following her father around, either audiotape player or paper and pencil in hand, trying to get as much wisdom (information) as possible.

Push Hands

By the time we got to the Shr Jung I had permission to push with any one, but still remained under Mort's guidance. I saw push hands as a game. When I was overcome, I let myself go, and was gracious about it. I pushed with many and some were better than I was, some were not.

Some had a sense of competition with me and most did not.

I chose to play with people who enjoyed the game, and valued the instruction from senior students and Professor as they occasionally passed by. However, when choices were limited, I would play with anyone, and play without injury or ego was not always possible.

This one guy who played with me insisted on pushing me hard into the wall. When he pushed, he caught me on the chest, and, because I was fairly stiff, I could not neutralize his push. He slammed me good and I landed hard against the wall. If I had not been a judo player, I might have been hurt. So, I asked him not to push with so much force. He said nothing, but he did it again, the very next push. I again asked him to take it easy. Again, no answer, and then he did it again. I told him one last time, with emphasis that this was not how I wanted to play. As he tried to do it again, I took one of his hands, which had found my upper chest, by the wrist, and lifted it, so his hand was over my shoulder. I then took his push. I added my body weight to the push and hurled myself backward to the wall, also pushing backwards with both of my legs. He made a fist before his hand hit the wall. He hurt his wrist, and split open his knuckles. I left his other hand on my chest and hit the wall hard, but because of the judo, I did not hurt myself. That was the only time anyone played rougher with me than I wanted to play. I am very happy that Professor did not see me doing that, because he might have misunderstood.

Let me explain: if Professor Cheng saw someone playing too rough, he would step in and teach the malefactor by pushing him the way he had been pushing, except stronger and better. He did this to give the person a taste of his own medicine. You could see some pretty good action watching those pushes, as the person went flying up and back like a rocket.

However, it is not the pushes that I was afraid of, but that Professor might have thought I was one of those rough guys who played to hurt people and not to learn. If so, he might not have liked me so much, and that would have hurt, beyond what any push could do.

I was a martial artist, I was ready to play with anyone, and be pushed by anyone who could. I came ready to set aside my ego as best as I could. But I did not come willing to be man handled because of the uncontrolled ego of a class mate.

If anyone complained that I was pushing too hard, as sometimes happened, I would soften my push. I did not want to hurt anyone. This was clearly not martial arts to me, as I had martial arts, and knew how to hurt someone without needing to resort to pushing anyone into a wall. This was just a game to me, to teach me how to relax, and to teach softness and listening skills thereafter. It still is today. While I know how it improves the martial arts, I still believe it is not necessary, correct, or desirable to hurt anyone in practice.

On the other hand, I learned a lot about push hands from a fellow student, who shall remain nameless. He knows who he is.

I pushed fairly stiffly when I played because I did not know any other way. I was softer then when I started, but not by much. I pushed hard, but not hard enough to hurt, just hard enough so that he would hit the wall with a satisfying slapping sound.

This player who I pushed with believed in "investing in loss." He intended to lose and did not see it as a path to learn to neutralize, and then overcome. I pushed with him often for a while. I pushed him into the wall, effortlessly, and repeatedly. He never did anything different, so I never did either. After a while, I learned that I could listen to his balance and just gently pop him into the wall; so I stopped pushing him blindly, with force. And so I learned a lesson in softness from this person who did not know he was teaching me, as he struggled with his own demons to "invest in loss."

Let me be clear here, "invest in loss" means to be soft. Not to resist force with force, but not to be pushed forever. If you are not learning a strategy to defeat the pushes, you are not investing properly.

A number of my classmates at the Association and the Shr Jung also pushed me, regularly and well. No one approached the techniques of the Professor, or to a lesser but still quite effective level, Stanley, Lou Kleinsmith, or Morty. Let me say here that Ed and Tam were soft, and much better than I was, but no memories come to mind of playing push hands with them. Though, I do remember sword dueling with Tam (details later).

Also, I did not push with Maggie. In my pride, I thought I could beat her, and so I did not think playing her would have been a learning experience. Also, I was no bully. So my only thought about Maggie and push hands was that I would have wanted to protect her if, in Professor's absence, someone was giving her a hard time. From my perspective, on this side of life, I do not know if I could have beaten Maggie. She may very well have surprised me. But such are the ego decisions I made when I was young and strong. I have no regrets about feeling protective towards Maggie.

Pushing with Professor

I got my best lessons from the Professor himself. If I had not pushed with him, and if he had not been so soft, I would never have known what to strive for. I do not know how many others had these types of experiences. I do know that some did not. They experienced Professor as a ten-ton truck. My pushing experiences were lessons, intended for me. He was a role model of what softness was, and how to win effortlessly. Though it was years before I was able to develop and use his methods, even in the less than optimal way that I do.

Pushing with Professor had two sides to it. There were the times when he neutralized, and the times when he pushed. And like two sides of the same coin, they were very different.

The feeling of being neutralized by Professor was that he was very empty and I flew by as he neutralized to the nth degree and I fell over, essentially, myself. When I had pushed him so far that I thought I had to lean on him, he just was not there to be leaned on. He appeared to be an optical illusion.

One time I pushed him straight back as far as I could push forward without falling. He sat straight back in, and then over, his rear leg without stepping and smiled at me. Then I pushed him to the side where he had no rear foot, at ninety degrees to the first push. He again, went effortlessly to the side. Now he was even further off his center. He smiled at me. At that point he touched me behind my rear shoulder, lightly, and I fell over and bounced away, without any force from him at all.

From this kind of push hands, I saw an example of this soft ability to root, and the softness of his body and hands, and his leg strength and balance. I also saw his ability to sense my balance and with a very light touch, off-balance me and send me hopping into a corner.

Another point I would like to make about his softness: He wore a carefully pressed traditional Chinese knee-length kind of shirt, or perhaps you could call it a short robe. It was immaculately pressed. When he presented his arm to be pushed, I could push as slowly or as violently fast as I chose. I could not make the crease of the robe, which kind of flopped over his arm towards my hand, touch the skin of his arm. I have never met anyone else who could be so soft. He was that light, that soft.

Being pushed by Professor was a very different thing, and I do not consider the light touches he gave me to send me flying when he was neutralizing as pushes. When he was demonstrating, or for film, he did something very different from what he did with me. When he pushed for film, people went flying back and could not get their legs under them. Even when he pushed me, and he did not add that kind of "chi", like when he demonstrated, he still sent me flying.

He sat in a stance before me as I sat in one before him. Then, he just touched me. I sensed him settle in, and I felt a sense of electricity, a charge at the point where my arm was being lightly touched, where it was in physical contact with his hands. And I just took off. It appeared to me that I was moving in slow motion. My ears worked, but sound had that distant echoing quality, like I was under water.

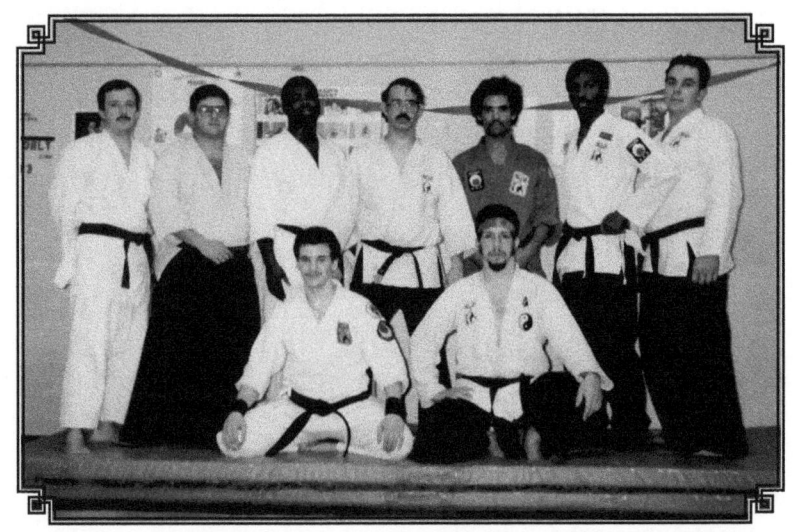

Patience T'ai Chi teaching staff, 1987. From left: Tony Botan, Eric Schneiderman, Cirilo Smith, William C Phillips, Ricard Perpignand, Roosevelt Moore, and Arnold Lenkersdorf

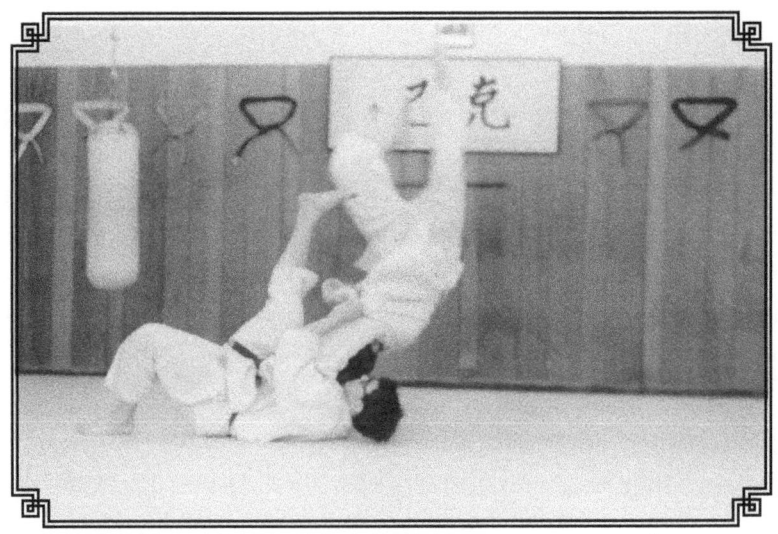

William C. Phillips performs *tomonage* at the Bay Ridge Dojo.

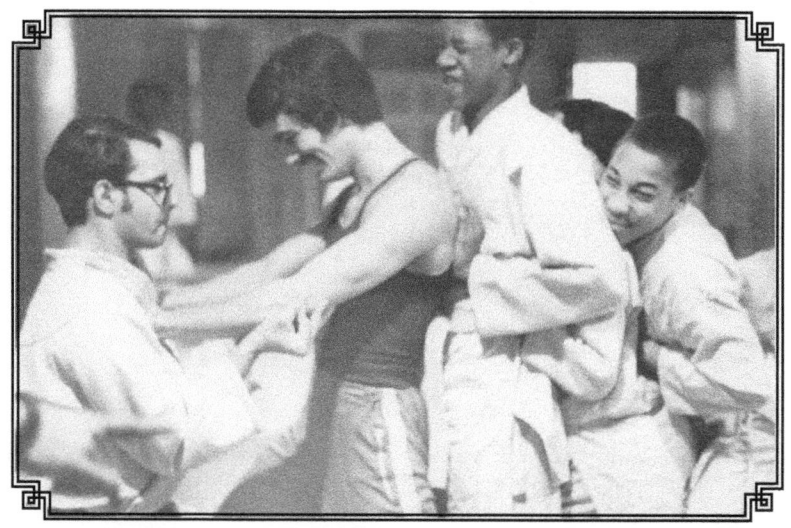

Demonstration of a foothold technique with students at the Patience T'ai Chi Association in Boro Park (second location).

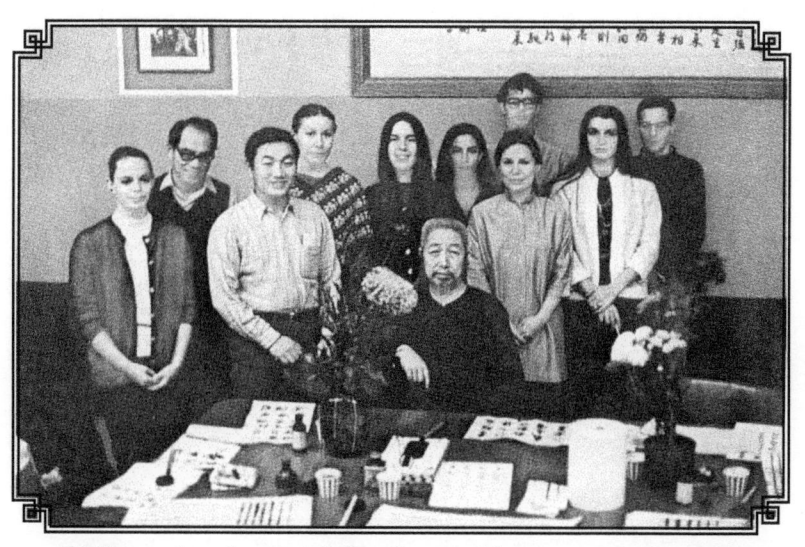

Calligraphy class with Professor Cheng, summer 1970. The author stands at the rear. *Photo credit:* Ken Van Sickle

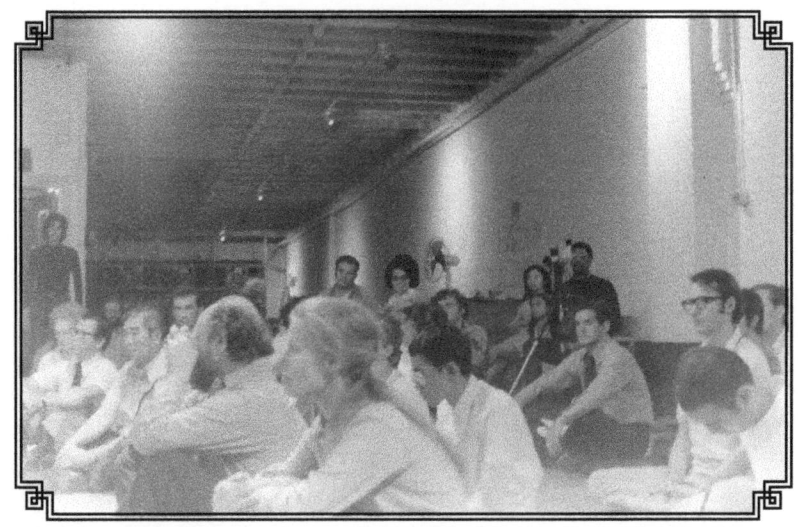

Students at the Shr Jung School Of Culture And The Arts. In the foreground is senior student Maggie Newman.

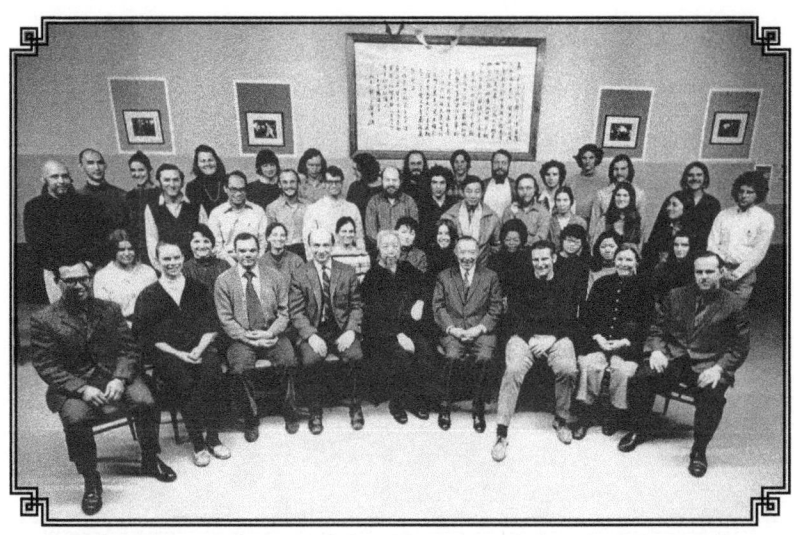

An early 70s era photo of the Shr Jung School with Professor Cheng Man-Ch'ing and his students. The author stands in the third row (first row standing) to the left of Professor Cheng. *Photo credit:* Kenneth Van Sickle

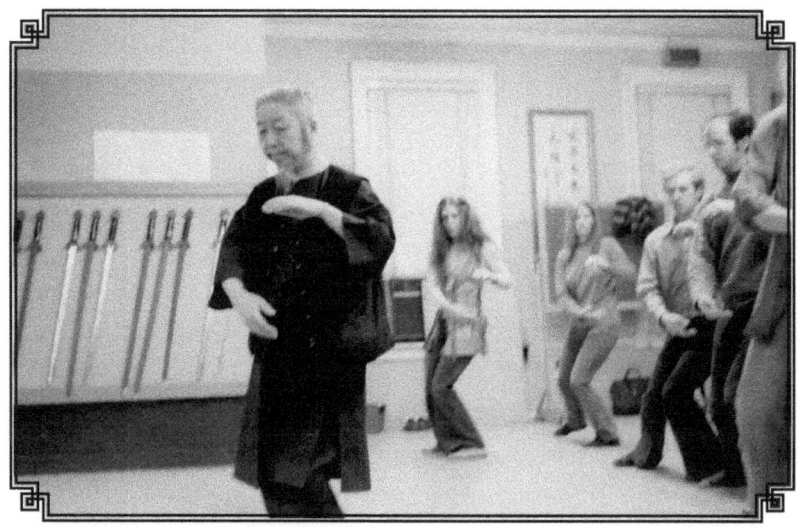

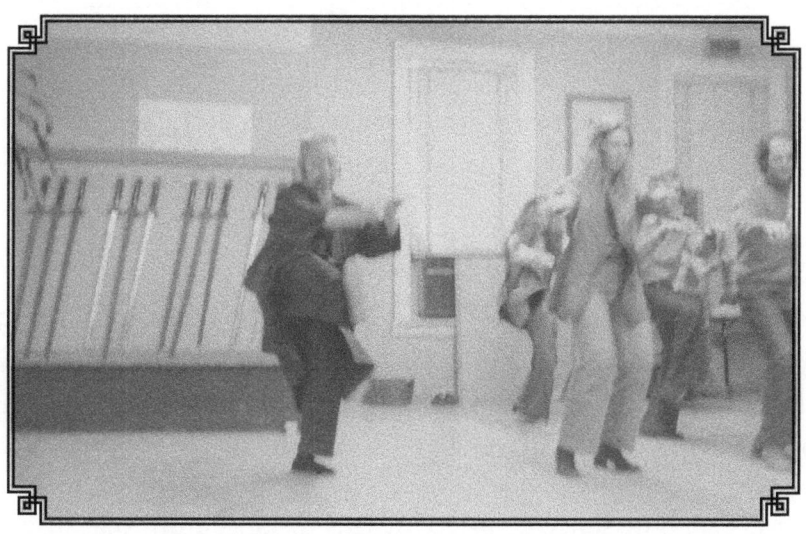

Professor Cheng teaches form correction at the Association.

Professor Cheng teaches form correction at the Association.

He took my wrist in his hand as my arm straightened slowly, like a slack rope held firmly on one end, playing out slowly as I rose. When I got to the end of the flexibility in my arm, the rope taut, I stopped perceiving that I was moving in slow motion. I suddenly noticed that I was moving at what felt like 60 miles an hour at an up angle of about 45 degrees. I shook violently as my arm, once the slack had played out, took the shock of the push. Then my hearing came back.

This was my experience of Professor's push. It was soft, yet very powerful, very very powerful. His contact with my arm was barely perceptible, yet his push was electric. And his push was irresistible.

I have said this before, to all who would listen: I know that people had different experiences with Professor Cheng. Many were pushed very differently, more like his filmed pushes. However, if Professor wanted to be soft, I suspect they would have had little more to feel than I did. But when Professor wanted to be hard, he gave them an unpushable something to try to push. He had a terrific root. He could send any one flying, the hard way, as well as the easy way.

I believe he had his reasons for everything he did and for the way he played every one that he played.

I have gotten some little bit of the softness of Professor, and you can see it, and feel it in me. I do not have much of the pushing ability that he had. It would be fun just to experience it once more, if I could.

Sword Dueling

Professor wanted us to play push hands and duel softly. In fact, for dueling, he would put aluminum foil on the swords so that if you made too much contact, as students dueled with each other, the foil would rip and you could clearly see that too much pressure was being applied to the sword. You cannot really see in the DVDs how softly he played at this distance from that magical time. However, there is one piece of evidence you can see. When Professor died, his shoes and his sword were placed in a display case. You could clearly see that the aluminum foil wrapping his sword was fresh and like new, completely unsullied by pressure. Consider the pressure that his students, including me, tried to put on his sword. Not only could we not put pressure on his sword, we could not get the damned thing out of our faces, or away from our bodies. Professor's sword point was almost always in your face or threatening your body when you dueled with him. You could not take his sword away, except by quitting the match. I could not put pressure on Professor's sword and I could not put pressure on the man. I was not the only one. All of us were roundly defeated by the Professor.

The two best that I dueled with were Professor Cheng and Tam. Tam was so soft, and I was so stiff. I was not much of a work out for him, except as an example of what not to do. He was a lot softer than me, and I could not stick him, or slice him. Tam could stick and slice me at will, and was quite polite in not doing so, stopping his sword short of my body, or running his sword gently in front of me. We both knew he won. He felt no need to rub it in.

While a sword in Tam's hand was very soft, Professor's sword was like smoke. The tip pointed at me and the hilt was in his hand. I could push his sword out of my way, and at the end of my move, the point of the sword was still staring me in the face. His hand with the hilt of the sword, was off to the side, where I apparently had pushed it. I could then push it the other way, and still, there it was, the sword tip, in my face. I had no sense of resistance as I pushed, it just went, which is why I characterize it as having the quality of smoke. Today you might characterize it as a hologram. Professor's sword just did not feel as if it were there. If I retreated, he advanced, with nothing to feel, and I did not advance as the sword point discouraged moving in that direction. But the tip was always staring me in the face, six inches away, followed by the rest of his gleaming unsullied sword. Through it all, Professor was always smiling at me, this beautiful angelic smile. You can see an example of that smile on the cover of this book and on my DVDs. I took a picture of him smiling his beautiful smile at me.

Not everyone was as soft or as considerate as Professor, but fortunately they were wooden swords, so no one was seriously hurt. Though, in mute testimony, the aluminum foil on the students' swords were all chipped, holed and ripped.

Like his students, Professor's sword was wrapped with the same foil. Unlike the students, his sword was completely unscathed. It shined, with no blemish. Such was the quality of his dueling.

I get a pair of swords of my own

Professor asked a number of us if we wanted to get swords. Of course we did. We were measured for the swords, from our tan t'iens to the floor, and then the swords were sent for. They were ordered from Taiwan and delivered by ship and so it took a while for the swords to arrive. I bought a wooden sword for eight dollars and a real sword for forty dollars, which was a lot of money at the time.

I did not wrap my wooden sword in aluminum foil. It would not have been clean and unripped very long in that state if I had. I had a long way to go to become soft enough not to scrape off the aluminum foil when I dueled. I do not know if I could do it, even now.

We were expected to treat the sword as if it was very heavy as we did our sword form, though in reality the wooden swords were quite light. We were told, I think by Lou, that real swords in ancient China were very heavy if they were made to be strong. This was because the Chinese did not have the superior metallurgy that the Japanese had used in making the Samurai sword. So the Chinese swords were heavy and they still broke in the heat of battle. This is why folklore grew up about swordsmen always looking for "magical" swords that were light and strong and would not break in a sword fight. Those swords would confer victory on their owners. While in reality they might not confer victory, they would confer a level of mobility and speed upon its user because of the lightness of the sword. Hence, the wielder of that sword had a much greater chance of victory.

Anyway, practicing with a light wooden sword, we were to imagine and treat the sword as if it were heavy. Push and then follow. This would also give us the sensitivity to play lightly, and bring our ch'i up to the point of our swords. Doing so would help us to lightly feel our partners ch'i and win the duel. In this sense it aids in push hands as well, because after learning to be sensitive all the way down your arm, to your fingers, and then to the tip of your sword, it is much easier to be sensitive down your arm and just to the tips of your fingers.

I have since "borrowed" my senior student Jim Leporati's 25-pound metal sword to teach the opening moves of the sword form. If the sword is heavy, you can get a feel of it, and then transfer the feel back into a lighter sword. With Jimmy's sword, unless you are very strong, it will break your wrist if you try to hold it in the air, as you perform some of the postures very slowly. This is not the case with the light wooden sword. To make an analogy, it is like learning to listen to a scream, so that you know what sound is, so that you can eventually learn to listen for a whisper.

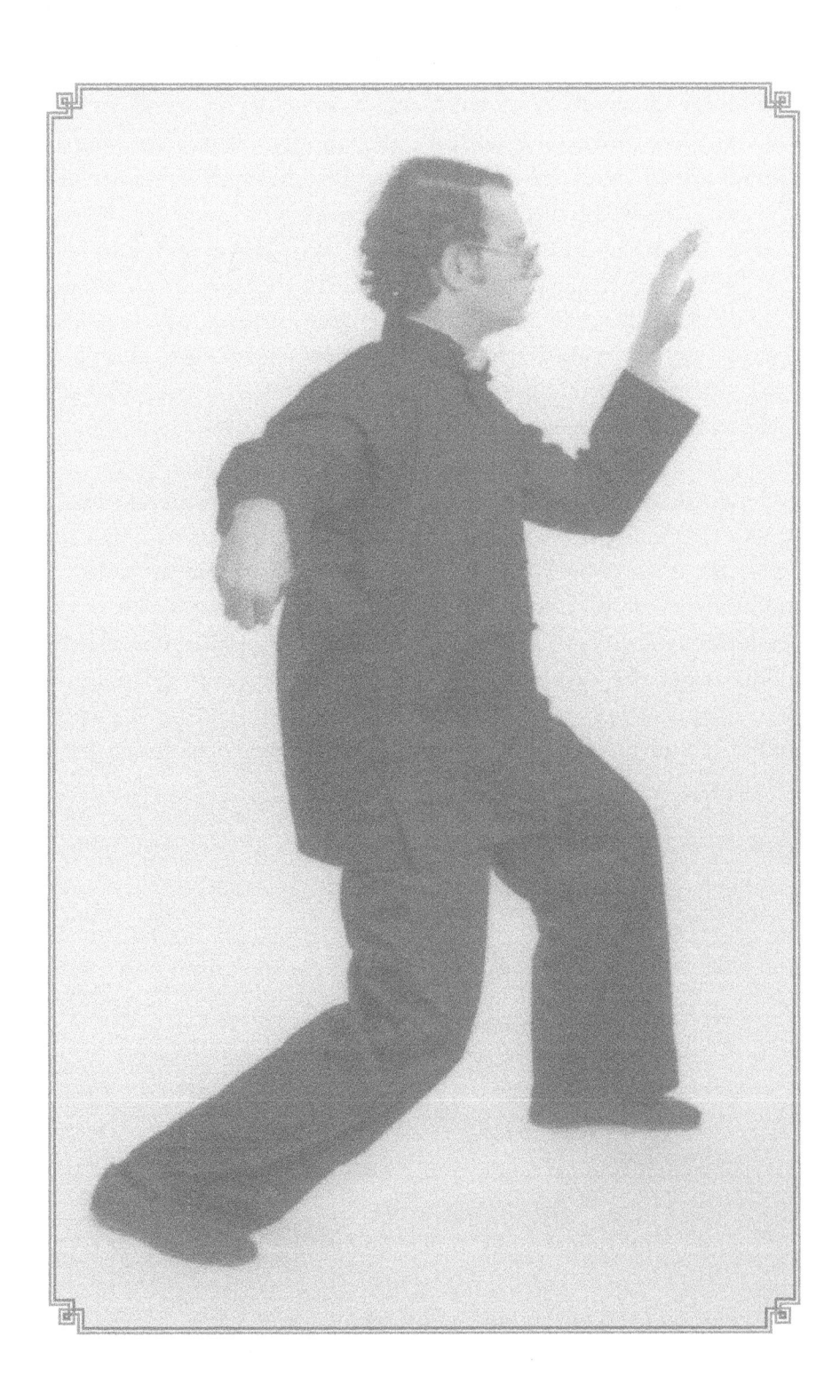

Chapter 8

More Stories from the Shr Jung

Professor Cheng meets an unexpected challenge

There was a student who challenged Professor Cheng. We were stunned that one of our number would do such a thing. That Professor Cheng had great skill was a matter not of faith, but of experience, our experience. He had proved himself to us, time and again, in ways of his own choosing. So we thought it was quite disrespectful for any one of us, his students, to actually challenge him. However, Professor Cheng handled the situation with calm and with dignity.

Professor held out his hand and said that if that person could turn his palm over, he would never call himself Cheng Man-Ch'ing again. Professor Cheng then put a white tissue or piece of handkerchief on his hand and offered it to the challenger. The challenger took Professor Cheng's hand, almost like shaking hands, except that the Professors hand was on top, and the challengers on the bottom. The two of them stepped around each other, a little like ba gua, stepping around the room, gripped hand in hand. The challenger, young and strong, trying to turn Professor Cheng's hand, the Professor holding his hand steady through it all. After about two minutes, though it seemed a lot longer than that, the challenger found no success in this exercise and admitted defeat.

Round one to Professor Cheng

The challenge was not over. For a second challenge, the challenger wondered out loud if he could hit Professor Cheng. He asked if Professor Cheng would be able to take the blows. The Professor let him try. Professor Cheng took a deep stance and the challenger threw a very strong reverse punch and then another and then a couple more. These punches were from the floor and through his hips at Professor Cheng's body. The challenger's waist was turning and his weight shifting and his legs were straining into these powerful punches. You could hear the punches thumping in as they landed, so heavy were those punches. Professor Cheng took the punches without neutralizing, though he could easily have turned and let each punch go harmlessly by. That would have been skill enough for us. Instead, Professor Cheng was like a solid wall, and as the punches thudded into Professor's abdomen, they had no apparent effect.

Round two to Professor Cheng

Still not giving up, our errant classmate wanted to challenge Professor Cheng to a fight. He was not happy with the palm challenge. He was not convinced by Professor's taking a few punches, though powerfully delivered, in spite of the fact that the punching was his own idea.

So Professor Cheng accepted that as well. They started, and the Professor attacked, his hands were constantly in the challenger's face and body; the challenger could not come even close to blocking the Professor. Finally, backed up against a wall, with Professor Cheng's hands lightly striking in front of his eyes: on his throat, solar plexus, and testicles, our challenger classmate realized that he had lost. At this time the challenge was over, and the challenger had to admit defeat.

IN THE PRESENCE OF CHENG MAN-CH'ING

Final round to Professor Cheng as well

This was an amazing feat if you think about it. Professor Cheng was in his 70s and his challenger was a healthy young man in his 30s who had studied martial arts. Yet Professor Cheng beat him handily, with a calm and collectedness that you expect to see in kung fu challenges in the movies.

At a talk in the school some time later, we got a lesson in Chinese manners as well. Professor Cheng asked us why no one stepped up to take the challenge for him. I was shocked. It never occurred to me. If that was what was supposed to have happened, I was sorry, because I respected Professor Cheng greatly and loved him as a father figure as well. I would gladly have stepped in if I had known that it was appropriate, even perhaps expected. I just did not think it was my place to do so. I had no idea what the protocol was in this situation, or even that there was any. For all I knew, anyone trying to intervene would have been insulting the Professor, representing the Professor with a lot less skill than Professor Cheng had. However, what Professor Cheng did was a lesson to all who were present. No one of us could have defeated the challenger so convincingly, and many not at all. No one of us could have had the effect that Professor had, of showing his martial superiority over all, in a calm and relaxed way. On the day of the challenge, he was truly the best.

My second major embarrassment: Mr. mouse story

I was studying Chinese as I wanted to be able to speak to Professor in his own language, and not through an interpreter. To aid in this endeavor, I went to the Chinese movies, where there were subtitles in both English and Chinese, while the spoken language was Mandarin, which was what Professor spoke. I was developing a spoken and a written vocabulary.

As I have noted already, I knew that one rendering of "Ni

how mah" was, "How are you?", while another was "You good horse", depending on the tones you used as you said the words. There are four tones in Mandarin. But I was never sure I was not saying, "You good horse," instead of "You well<interrogative>" So I had settled on the vernacular, "How bu how," (well not well) for how are you. I thought there was less opportunity to get it wrong if I kept it simple.

I was not aware, exactly aware, of the word for teacher. I thought Lao Tsu was teacher. After all, we had studied the work of Lao Tsu the philosopher or wise teacher, so I thought.

So I went up to him one day, and said, "Lao Tsu, how bu how." He looked at me, sharply at first, then surprised and a bit confused. He was looking at me like he was not sure what he had heard. I repeated, "Lao Tsu, how bu how." Finally, he broke into a broad grin and he said, pointing at himself, "How, how, Cheng how," and then he walked away, smiling and shaking his head. As if he could not believe it, in a funny way.

I was confused. Boy was I confused. What could I have said to have gotten that reaction? I walked up to Ed Young and told him about the interaction. He asked what I had said, and when I told him, he nearly fell out of his seat laughing. He would not tell me what I had actually said. I wanted to know. The same thing happened when I told Tam. He convulsed with laughter, and Tam was very serious and almost never laughed. Morty's wife was also caught in a spasm of laughter. This was uncharacteristic for her, to not at least tell me what I had said that was so funny. For about half an hour, a very frustrating half an hour, the story spread, and as people heard what I had said, and looked over their shoulders at me and turned away, peals of laughter broke out spontaneously again and again. Finally, someone was willing to tell me what I had done. I had called Professor a mouse (with my ignorance, mispronunciation and tone). I had said to him, "Mouse, how are you?" I was so embarrassed I wanted to hide under the table, but he seemed to take it with good humor.

I learned later that the word for teacher was Lao Shr.

City University with Patrick and Wayne

I do not remember the exact year, but Patrick and Wayne Cheng were doing a demonstration of T'ai Chi at a China Night at the Graduate Center of the City University of New York. I believe it was on 34th Street in New York City at that time. I volunteered to help, as did a classmate from the Shr Jung. We had a wonderful time, and pictures are included here. We, the helpers, did form and push hands while Patrick and Wayne narrated and explained.

Open Strike Over His Shoulder

I was curious to see how Professor would handle the speed of an open snap strike, but I did not wish to be disrespectful or to chance losing his affection for me. One day I approached him with respect and asked if I could throw an open snap strike over his shoulder. He indicated, through translation, to go ahead. I threw it over his shoulder so as not to hurt him in case I could hit him. No worries on that account. His hand met mine and rode with it to its end, as the hand snapped out, and he did not lose it. Then, at the end of its range, it started quickly back, and he still did not lose it. He was touching me from the start to the finish, and at no time, in spite of my quick reversal in speed, did he lose the hand. The pressure was light and even. He then smiled and walked away.

Years later, Zhang Lu–Ping, upon seeing my open snap strike, asked me where I had learned my Chen style. I informed him that I had not learned Chen, ever, but I had studied ju jitsu and learned or figured out how make snappy powerful moves. I moved with power from the legs and hips.

The open snap strike is, in itself, a story. In my ju jitsu class I saw Stan Israel do an open snap block once, just once, and I asked him how he did it. He said it was not that simple and walked away, of course. So I figured out how to do open snap block by myself. Then I figured out exercises to teach it. From there I figured out open snap strike, and the rest was history, as they say. I was able to hit anyone with it, almost at will. I sometimes set it up by feigning an opening to my stomach, but took the power out of any trading of blows by hitting the head, slightly before, hard, so there was no power in any incoming strike.

I would not have wanted to face a young me on the way up. And I was only sixty when I wrote this part of the story. How long will this book take in coming, I am seventy and still editing. Professor in his seventies was able to handle me with ease, Such was his softness and skill. He had told us if we were sexually moderate, we could hang on to what strength and power we had. I guess he was very moderate, as well as very skilled. At seventy I like to think I have some skill, but I am not up to facing strong youngsters. Perhaps I was not so sexually moderate.

The Hudson River Museum

I was driving along north of New York City one day in the fall of 1973. I was looking at the leaves turning from green to yellow, orange, and red along the highway, and for the cultural sites to be found north of New York City. I found a museum off the Saw Mill River Parkway, and decided to go in and take a look. To my utter surprise, Professor Cheng was there and he was having an art exhibition. I took a place in the balcony and watched as he prepared to draw a picture in black ink on a huge piece of paper that was spread out on a large table in front of him. He was silent for a minute, quietly meditating. Then he began, and he did not take his brush from the paper as he drew the whole painting. I think it was a bamboo tree. He did not see me, and after his demonstration, I got back into my car and drove away. Back at the Shr Jung, he never said a word about this event. He was modest, I guess, and/or did not think we would have been interested. I was fascinated and in awe. They gave out a booklet commemorating the show. I have mine. So, while I may not remember exactly what day the event was held, I know the show was November 25th to December 9th, 1973.

The Professor's Art

Professor had done a Christmas card for UNICEF in 1965, and an ex-girlfriend had given me the card for Christmas, long before I knew of Professor, long before I was studying T'ai Chi. Unfortunately, she broke up with me badly, and I threw the card away. After I knew about Professor Cheng, I went hunting for that card, to no avail. It is almost the only old card from that time I ever threw away, and it was something I would have valued greatly. So I guess it was not meant to be.

Once, at Morty and Ling's house, Professor asked me if I'd like to commission a painting from him. It would cost $1,000. I was told that it could be sold for as much as $1,500 as soon as it was completed. Unfortunately, that was almost three months take home pay for me. My wife thought that I was spending more than enough on T'ai Chi lessons and would not have me spend scarce money on a painting. Later, in a conversation with Ken Van Sickle, I learned to my everlasting regret that if I had told him I admired his work, he might have given me one for free. Looking back I wish I had taken Professor up on his offer. I would have cherished that painting. I would never have sold it.

The Consulate Pieces

Professor was famous, and he was featured on two pieces put out by the Taiwanese consulate in New York City. The first was a martial arts piece. There was a picture of him in a snake creeps up (squatting single whip) posture right on the front page. The second was a calligraphy piece, on the back page, of him doing calligraphy.

I have both of the original pieces. I got them when I was his student and I heard of their existence. I went uptown to the consulate and saw that they had stacks of each of them, and so I took a few. I used to give them out to my students, but stopped when I ran low on them.

A Secret

Professor's grasp of English was kind of a secret. If I asked a simple question, privately, sometimes he would just say yes or no and not wait for it to go through translation. In his lifetime I would never had said a word about this, as he never used English in public.

It makes sense that he did not want any facility he might have had with English to be known. I think he thought it best for a translator to tell him what was meant as well as translate his words so there would be no misunderstanding. It also gave him time to think about the question for an extra minute, if he understood it in English, before translation. That way his answer might be better thought out. To this day many think he did not speak or understand English and I believe that is the way he wanted it. So yes, confidentially, he spoke, or at least understood, some English, but for all public purposes he only spoke through a translator. Now that he is long gone from us, I do not think it hurts to let it be known.

This is something you should understand. It is not an easy skill to be able to answer on the spot. To this day, I would much rather answer in writing than orally. This is because the time it takes me to think it over and write an answer can mean the difference between answering badly and answering well. He had to think on his feet, and get it right the first time. It is a rare skill that does not get the benefit of reflection or an edit.

Professor's Energy in the Room

I always knew if Professor was at the Shr Jung. His energy lit it up. I felt him as a gentle loving presence in the room and I could tell if he was there or not just by poking my head in the door. If the place felt vacant, even if crowded, he was not there. If it felt warm and full, even if it was relatively empty, then he was there. Unfortunately, not many people experienced this.

Of tea and time with Professor

One stifling hot humid summer's day, when we could not practice any more due to the heat, he made a hot tea for us to drink. He said it was a cooling tea. Then, as we sipped it, he sat us down and gave a talk. Though it was very hot and sticky, gradually the heat and humidity faded away. At the time I was surprised, as I usually only found relief from the heat in air-conditioning or a cold drink. I remember still the sounds of the window fans, droning endlessly, and the cars' horns far below, on the Bowery, on Canal Street, fading gently away, as if they were coming from a different world, a different time. They were the only sounds we could hear when Professor was not speaking. The tea worked. I do not remember what he spoke about that day, only the wonderful feeling of the experience.

Another curious thing about that magical day: The hour we spent with Professor when he gave that summer talk went slowly. Usually when I was enjoying something the time just flew by. But not this day. Perhaps we were sharing his consciousness. It was a great pleasure, but the hour went by slowly, so slowly. I very much enjoyed that length of time. I was able to savor it, unlike most of the rest of my life.

I begin to teach T'ai Chi

First let me say, to be honest, that I had been teaching T'ai Chi, unauthorized, since I started at the Association, as I had three years instruction with Stanley. In the beginning I taught my ju jitsu and karate students secretly, as part of their instruction, one night a week.

While at the Shr Jung, I got permission to assist teaching T'ai Chi and an assignment to drive Ed Young and Herman Kauz to Connecticut to do so.

I picked up Ed and Herman in Manhattan, on West End

Avenue around 100th Street. When we got to Connecticut, I stayed with Ed and assisted him as he taught at the Yale T'ai Chi Club. Herman borrowed my car and went on to another location. It was the only time I ever loaned out my car that I was not nervous about it. Herman rejoined us when he was finished, and I drove us back to the city. I dropped Ed and Herman off and then went home, and to bed, as I had to rise early to go to work the next day.

This was my first official assistant T'ai Chi teaching experience. I was new to teaching outside of my own school, in public, so to speak, and took it way too seriously. As an example, I corrected this one woman by putting her thumb down when it was stuck up by tension. It would pop up again and, as I passed by, I would correct it down again. It was my job to walk up and down the rows of students, correcting, as Ed was teaching from the front. I probably corrected her a dozen times in the course of a single hour. In retrospect, I probably drove the poor woman right out of T'ai Chi.

I learned two things about teaching T'ai Chi in that class that affected my teaching style for years to come. First, teaching is like sculpture: rough out the big parts the first time through, and then do ever finer work in various and continued correction over time. Some people can learn without this process, and it is important to recognize them and teach them more of the details the first time. This is because they can learn them, and also because you do not want to bore them. But most people cannot learn too many details at one time and need to undergo this process. Second, if someone cannot do something, physically cannot, like the woman I mentioned above, even if it is just that the person is mentally not ready to see it, correcting again and again will not help. It will make the student self-conscious and not likely to continue. So, correct it once and let it go. Let them know, if they can understand it, what they need to do. That is enough. Remember to compliment them where they are, wherever they are, whatever they are doing, as long as they are trying. And compliment them for knowing where they eventually have to go.

Casual students need to have a good time as well as have a learning experience. They need to feel good about themselves, so they will stay long enough to benefit.

I Teach at the Shr Jung

Professor made me a teacher at the Shr Jung before he left for Taiwan that last time. As a result, I had a beginners' class on Sundays in the front of the Shr Jung by the windows facing the Bowery. I was both proud of myself and eager to do the best job I could.

Ed Young was teaching an advanced class in the middle of the Shr Jung, in front of the mirrors. When I was not sure of something, or had been asked a question I did not know the answer to, I would stop my class. I would walk over to Ed's class, and stand and wait respectfully to get Ed's attention. Then I would ask him. With his answer I would return to my class and teach it as it had just been explained to me.

One day Ed caught me in the men's room and said to me, "Bill, just teach, and answer questions as they come up. Then, if you have doubts about what you are teaching, or are not sure of the answers to some of the questions you get asked, come and ask me at some time when we are not teaching. I will answer you and then you can correct yourself at the next class meeting. Students will probably not remember what you taught or said the previous week, so you may not even have to acknowledge it if you were wrong." Ed was very tactful not to say it, but in my desire to get everything exactly right, I was interrupting both our classes with my questions.

So I learned to seem to be self-confident when I was teaching, whether I actually was or was not. That was a wonderful piece of advice for two reasons: First, as Ed had indicated, it was good to not be interrupting our two classes. It was also great advice because students want a teacher who is sure of himself, rather than one who is always checking his information. So much is "bedside manner."

I was the youngest teacher in Professor Cheng's school, both in age and in seniority. I did not realize this until later. Maybe I did not realize this at all, but Avi Schneier, a senior student of mine, pointed it out to me, in response to a story I was telling about the Shr Jung.

Maggie's Class

When Professor was away, that last time, Maggie ran an advanced class. She ran the class by asking us to make teaching contributions. Weekly, she selected several of us and asked us to show what we had learned. This way we could each benefit by what our classmates had gleaned from the classes.

Perhaps she wanted to get our perspectives on what we had learned, or maybe she was being gracious enough to let us show off what we had learned. In any case, this is how she ran that class. I thought it was very brave of her, to explore this method.

When it was my turn, I showed foothold, or rooting technique. I held the whole class, and then I tried to teach them how to do it. Unfortunately, they could not learn it. I thought they were soft enough, and knew they could do the posture for it. But they were not relaxed enough to learn to be essentially one relaxed, connected body, in order to do it themselves.

I should point out here that I may not have had the skill so well myself. When I did it standing upright, with my spine 90 degrees to the earth and there were many people pushing me, I sometimes hurt the arch of my back foot. For days after, the arch would be sore. It was only when I learned to do the foothold technique with a slight forward tilt, as if doing the Yang Long form, that the foothold ceased to hurt. I would also like to point out that Professor appears to be doing it just that way in the picture on page 26 of Chinese *Boxing, Methods and Masters*, by Robert W. Smith.

Let me say that my shoulders were never near as relaxed as

was required to do the technique as Professor did it. So I did the technique differently. I did it with the first person's hands placed on my chest, with the next person directly behind the first one, their hands on his back, the third behind the second, etc. When I tried to do it as Professor did it, my arm would collapse to my chest, or my shoulder would tense. In either case I would go flying back.

Also, I might add that, as I was developing the skill, I kept my eyes closed and had a student tell the line of pushers when to push, adding one at a time. If I opened my eyes during the process, I immediately got nervous, as I observed the line pushing me. I could not believe I was holding them. The result was immediate. I was not holding them; I went flying backwards.

Some words about Professor Cheng's skills

Professor was considered to be a master of Five Excellences, a special title, reserved for those who were recognized as masters of painting, poetry, calligraphy, medicine, and T'ai Chi Ch'uan. He was also a master of philosophy, and I believe, of ethics, as well. He wanted so much to teach us how to be good human beings. That was what Chung-yung was about.

He said Lau Tzu class would teach us the ways of heaven and earth, and of course we all wanted this information. He said Confucius class was to teach us to be good human beings, and there was significantly less enthusiasm for that.

As mentioned before, Professor was a doctor of Chinese medicine. He told us that we each had a yin point and a yang point moving around our bodies. These points could be hit by someone who knew about this and how to do it, and it would be fatal.

Professor talked of the seasons. He said in the spring, the ch'i of heaven comes down and ch'i of earth comes up out of the ground. The two ch'is mix and in that combined energy field things in nature grow. In the summer those energy fields remain mixed. In the fall, the process begins to reverse itself, the ch'i of heaven rises off the planet and the ch'i of earth sinks back down, and the leaves stop being green. In the winter the energy fields are just weak. On the other side of the planet, they are doing the opposite.

To me, the way he describes it is like three coins. The earth in this example is a nickel, the ch'i of earth is a dime and the ch'i of heaven is a quarter. If the dime comes up on one side of the nickel, it is missing from the other. If the quarter is low on one side of the nickel, it is far away on the other. In spring and fall, the energy fields reverse.

Professor was modest

Professor Cheng was modest. At the time of my studies with Professor, I took advantage of being in Chinatown to buy Chinese language kung fu magazines because they sometimes had pictures of Bruce Lee in them. I noticed, much to my surprise, that Professor Cheng was also in some of them. He never said anything about being in Chinese or American magazines. Though he was occasionally the focus of a story in an American magazine, he was much more often the focus of a story in Chinese magazines. His every move seemed to be newsworthy. There is even a photo in a magazine of him visiting with the President of the USA, but he never made a big deal out of it. In fact, he never even mentioned it.

Professor the author

He did tell us about the books he wrote. Professor said he wrote so many books that if they were laid flat on the ground they would stack to his height. I was told much later, by Barbara Davis, that he was speaking metaphorically. However, he did write many books, including at least one book on gynecology. I do not know how many of his books were translated and published in English. In addition to what was published, there were notes distributed to students that would have been enough to have become a book on Lao Tsu and two on Confucius. I think one was the Great Learning, the other, Chung-yun. He also had a book on T'ai Chi and I Ching, and a couple just on T'ai Chi. I want to get and read the book on T'ai Chi and I Ching if it is ever available in English.

SOME MORE OF MY FOOD INCIDENTS

I used to pride myself that I could eat hot food, but it was only my ego talking. I guess, in retrospect, the food I ate was not very hot in those days. One day Mort and Ling took me to a restaurant on East Broadway. When I went out with them, Mort ordered for us all, including me. They had ordered some white cabbage looking stuff to be put on the table as an appetizer. I took some with my chopsticks, and ate it. It tasted good. Then the burning started, and it burned and burned. I drank my whole glass of water, and it still burned, so I drank Mort's water and then Ling's.

Mort and Ling laughed and laughed at me. It may have been a set up, as that cabbage, which tasted pretty good, was so very hot in my mouth after a bit. I felt the heat make the rounds in my intestines and then eventually felt something come out the other end, still a burning hot sensation. After that, I decided I would get into less trouble if I stopped eating, and bragging about eating, hot spicy foods. Nowadays, I can eat some hot foods, like kimchi or other Korean specialties, but I eat for the taste, and leave the burning, and the bragging, to others.

Another food story at that time, though not really about the food, was this: One day I went into a restaurant to eat lunch. I had my practice slippers with me, rope-soled Chinese shoes. I walked into the back of the place, sat at a table, and put the rope soles on the table next to me so I would not forget them. This alarmed the restaurant staff, who apparently thought I might have been making a statement about being a tough guy and/or not paying for the food. They talked among themselves and then one got on the telephone. Shortly after, a gang of tough young Chinese kids came and sat surrounding me, at three tables, one across, one in front and one across and in front. This helped the staff be more relaxed. I finished my meal, got the check, paid it, and left. The kids, who never had more than tea while I ate, followed me out of the restaurant and then disappeared into the crowd. It appeared that they were the restaurant's insurance.

Actually, I do not know why I was not at Sum Hey Rice Shop or Kam Bo Rice Shop at this time, as they were my restaurants of choice. Perhaps they came later. I was a regular at Sum Hey until the waiters there opened Kam Bo across the street and then I was a regular there. At Kam Bo they invited me to a free opening dinner celebration and put my picture on the wall. Unfortunately, it is not there anymore, I checked. But by then I had not eaten there for years.

As I said, I would often eat at Sum Hey and later on at Kam Bo. When I did, I would eat beef, tofu, bok choy, broccoli and onions on rice with sweet and sour sauce. It cost, at the time $1.25. They said no Chinese would ever eat that dish with that sauce. But I liked it, and since they were willing to prepare it, I ordered it and ate it.

After such meals I would return to the Shr Jung, and stay to hang out and play push hands with anyone who wanted to, until around five o'clock or so, when it was time to head home if it was a Sunday night. If I was on a school vacation I might join a group and go downstairs and eat some more Chinese food with them, or take in a sword or kung fu movie.

In those late Sunday evenings, people would be practicing calligraphy by the table in the back, and some tea might be available as well.

Professor Passes On

Professor gave an informal talk before he left for Taiwan. He was telling us he would not be around as long as we thought. He told us that we were holding T'ai Chi here in New York City because we wanted to study with him. He demonstrated a closed fist to show the image, of holding T'ai Chi in. He said it was like a flower holding onto its seeds. He went on to say that when he passed away, T'ai Chi would spread to the four corners of the USA. To continue with this image, he opened his hand, and said, "Letting the seeds get taken by the winds." As long as he was alive and coming back to New York, T'ai Chi would stay bottled up here in New York.

We heard that, while on this, his last visit to Taiwan, when Tam lost Professor's passport and he could not return easily to New York, he was not upset. He seemed to think it was fine.

When Professor died, we in New York were in shock. We just could not understand it. He seemed so youthful and healthy and vibrant. We were informed by a telegram, which was then put in the display case for all to see. As the shock passed and we really started to miss him, we gathered ourselves and had a memorial. Robert W. Smith came up from Washington DC and Ben Lo came from somewhere as well. Others also came. There were people I did not know, and there was no easy way to know who they may have been, as no one was banging their own drum on that solemn occasion. I did know many of the people, and took a couple of pictures of them.

His shoes and sword were placed in the display case when he left us. It was so sad to look at them and know he was gone.

WILLIAM C. PHILLIPS

I CONTINUE ON MY LIFE PATH

After Professor passed, I continued to study. After the school broke up I went to Mort's and Ling's house for additional private instruction. After that, I studied and practiced alone, until in 1988 I met Zhang Lu–Ping. I had ten years with him, and in 1998, when he passed, I started to study alone again. I am what I have become as a result of all that.

A dear friend, Master Jou Tsung Hwa, told me that the form could teach me. At the time I protested. I did not believe it. Besides, I had been, and then was, under the instruction of masters. I was just too young to understand. Now I do, old friend. The form has taught me, and continues to teach me. Great teachers laid the foundation, and practice is the catalyst. The form is my last great teacher.

THE VOTING ORGANIZATION

It is not my intention to talk of the animosity of the breakup of the school after Professor's death. There were many hard feelings, as bad decisions were made by a couple of people who should have known better. They have since passed away, and it is not good to remember people by their worst selves and actions, but by their better selves and actions. I, for one, would be happy to let their actions be lost to history. But the breakup did happen, and its effect helped to make us what we became. So, this is the outline of some of the facts, just the facts, without the arguments or the emotions.

This last time, as Professor prepared to depart for Taiwan, his mind went to our governing ourselves in his absence. It gives credence to my belief that he knew he was not coming back and wanted to leave the school in good hands. Or you could make the argument that he remembered what happened at the Association and wanted to leave us prepared to take independent action on our own.

In any case, Professor Cheng set up an organization to run

the school in his absence. He had never done this before, though he had been away before. That, and his comment that after his lifetime his T'ai Chi would spread, had me wondering, but he was so healthy and vibrant, no one gave more than a passing thought to his leaving us that way.

In this organization, the senior six, the inner ring, had one vote each. The next twelve, the middle ring, had one-half vote, apiece. The outer ring, of eighteen, had no vote at all, but got to attend meetings and voice their opinions at those meetings. I was a member of this third group, and I was there at the first and only meeting.

The landlord had offered to sell us the building where the Shr Jung was (87 Bowery). He offered it at a huge discount, it was said, because he believed in what we were doing. Every one voted yes to buy the building, except two people. Every one spoke in favor of it, except for those same two people. They were out voted, but they said they owned the corporation of the Shr Jung, and that we worked for them, so the other votes did not count.

In fact they did own a corporation, which they set up when we were on Crosby Street, after the problem with the Association. They had set it up to deposit the money collected as T'ai Chi dues, so that the IRS would not think they had another source of income. That was its main purpose. It was not supposed to confer ownership of the school.

When we heard this, I and almost everyone else walked out, and that is all I have to say about it.

When, many years later, I ran the event The Celebration of the 100th Anniversary of the Birth of Professor Cheng Man-Ch'ing, it was for the purpose of commemorating his birthday. It was also for the purpose of trying to bring all of us together, the student family of the Professor. There were also the students of the students, in New York City, who had remained loyal to the family and those who had not. There were branches of other senior people who were teaching all over the country, who we did not know as well as we should. By having students of many branches as teachers and welcome guests, we made a big step forward in reuniting ourselves. CMC (Cheng Man–Ch'ing) celebrities Maggie Newman and William C. C. Chen and his family were in attendance. The event was presided over by Katy and Ellen Cheng, Professor's daughters.

We are all one family: the Professor's family.

IN THE PRESENCE OF CHENG MAN-CH'ING

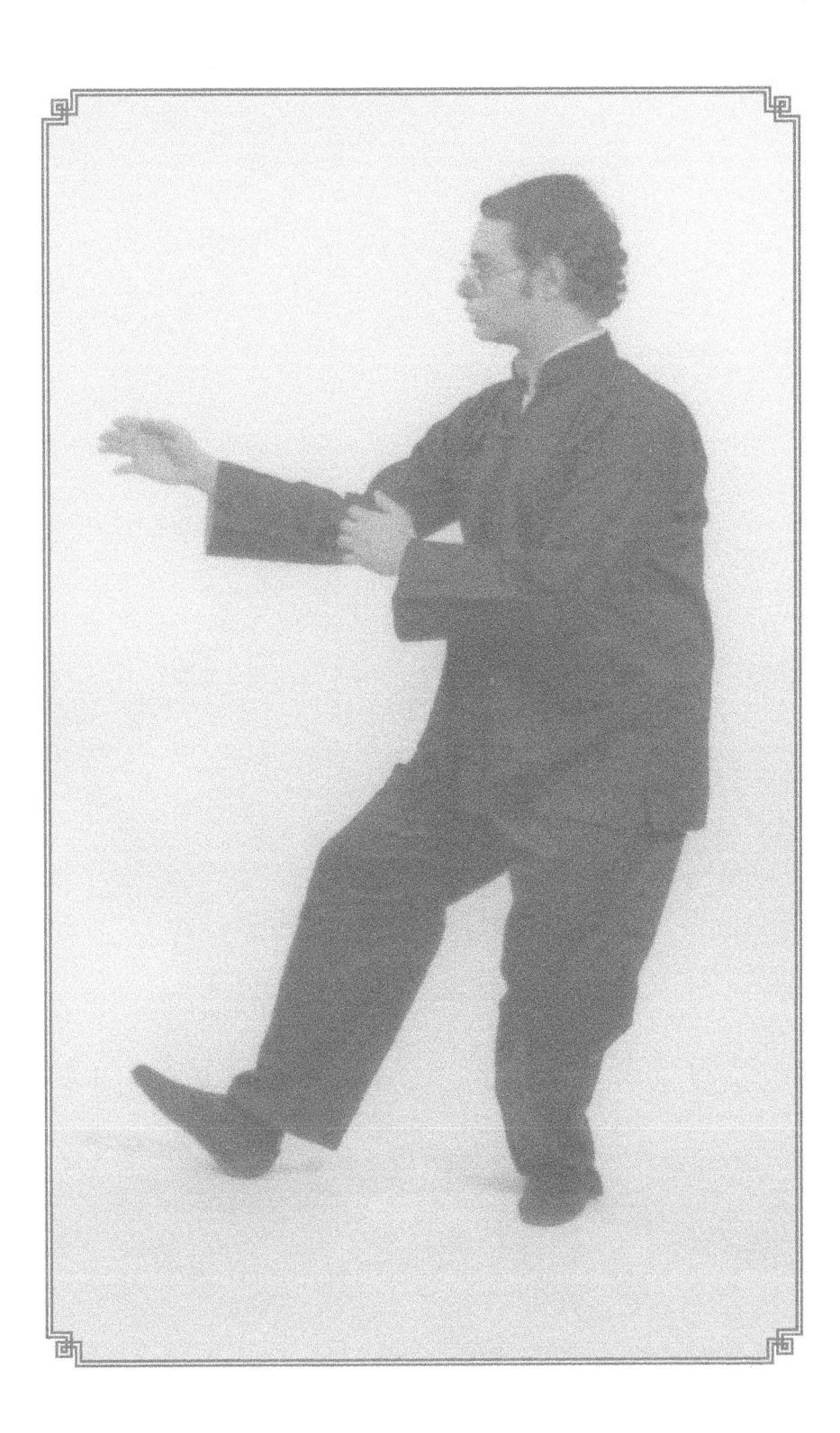

Chapter 9

Some Reflections on the Senior Students

Morton Raphael, a lifetime of friendship

Mort was one of Professor's senior students. Mort could make me fly lightly, or blast me, like Stanley, or, toy with me, like Lou, but did not often play me with multiple break balances, as Lou often did. I knew Mort best at the school because Professor Cheng assigned Mort as a mentor to me when I finally got permission to go on to push hands. I did not realize it at the time, but again, Professor Cheng singled me out for special treatment. Everybody did not get a mentor. In fact, I do not know of anyone else that was given a mentor in Professor Cheng's school. While there might have been, I am not aware of it.

Mort came to Professor's school with a background in judo and aikido, and he became really good at push hands. He was quiet about his skill, and did not show off, so only those who played with him ever found out. I was so lucky that he was tasked by Professor Cheng with mentoring and teaching me. So, at the Association and at the Shr Jung, I played a lot with Mort, often an hour or more, two or three times a week. I was terminally stiff at the start of our time together and I would frustrate Mort to no end. But he cared. I know that because he continued to teach me no matter how stiff and difficult to teach I was.

I had been primarily trained in judo, ju jitsu, and karate. So

Mort and I were both martial artists, and that may have helped to give him some insights on what my problem was and how to work with me. When Stanley taught me T'ai Chi, he did not give me any particular instruction about relaxing, and, fortunately, so I thought, I was very strong from my other martial training. As Mort worked with me, I became aware that being strong was not necessarily an advantage in T'ai Chi. I came to this understanding because Mort was drumming it into me that I had to somehow learn to not rely on that strength. Though at first, I had no clue as to how to do that.

I drove Mort to distraction as he tried to teach me to relax. This was because he taught me push hands by teaching me to relax, and I could never become relaxed enough to suit Mort. It was a process of years until I finally learned to relax, really relax. But I got there a little piece at a time, a very little piece at a time, every Thursday and Sunday. I would go to the school and Mort would do exercises with me that he designed to teach me to relax. Then he would play push hands with me. I would be pushed to the wall, time and again. Mort spent some time and ingenuity devising those exercises to try to teach me to relax, to neutralize, and to listen. But while he was making an impression on my mind, my body just seemed lesson-proof.

Let me explain it this way: I did not know the difference between relax and collapse. That more than anything else eventually drove Mort to some impatience with me, and he was a pretty patient guy. I was either collapsed or stiff from his perspective (and from the point of view of my understanding today, at this end of my training). From my perspective at the time, I was totally confused. I got him so frustrated with my lack of progress with this concept, of relaxed aliveness that he sometimes used to tweak my nose to let out that frustration when I continually did not get it. I always took it as a sign he liked me and cared about my T'ai Chi education. So I took the tweaking in good humor, and sometimes had to try very hard not to sneeze in his hand.

As I mentioned above, Mort designed a series of exercises for me as he tried to figure out how to get me to relax. I did learn something, if not the lesson Morty intended. I learned the lesson of teaching through exercises. At the time I was teaching judo, ju jitsu and karate as well as remedial reading in high school. The idea of teaching those things as well as push hands through exercises was an idea that I adopted, to help students improve, in both skill and understanding.

Mort tried to help me to learn and to have access to the best knowledge. He let me copy the personal corrections that he had written into his "green book" of form to further explain the text and pictures. It was a book that could be purchased at the school. (I later bought a bunch and, while they lasted, gave them to all my students who became teachers.) Mort gave me access to the audiotapes that were made before I was a student. His wife was my personal link to the Professor when Ed and Tam thought I was bothering and exhausting Professor with too many questions.

Mort introduced me to his nephew, Steven, and I practiced with him under Mort's tutelage and with correction, always correction. In addition to playing push hands with them I also played regular push hands with many of the rest of my classmates. However, I played mostly under Mort's supervision, with Mort telling me when I played improperly, or with too much strength.

When the school broke up, Mort stayed home in New Jersey, and practiced and taught a couple of students from there, privately, one at a time. I would go out to spend a day with Mort. We would practice and hang out in his wonderful back yard. His house was at the top of a hill, and the driveway was a steep challenge. But I remember fondly the sun of a beautiful summer's day showing through the leaves of the trees. Framed by the blue sky, some leaves were hit by the sun and were a bright green, others were in the shade and were a dark green. We trained and then sat in the shade and enjoyed the day with Mort's large dogs, who had the run of the property. (Mort had the property fenced in so the dogs could run free and not get out.) Then, as evening fell, we would go inside and eat the wonderful food that Ling Raphael had prepared.

I finished with my lessons at Mort's when Mort went to push me, and I was relaxed and nothing much happened. So he tried again, the same, and one last time, the same. That is when I knew I had learned. When nothing happened I knew I had learned what he had been trying to teach me for so long and with so much effort: to be soft and neutralize. Finally, I was relaxed enough to let a fast one inch or so push come and just sit in with it.

Let me say that Mort could still have pushed me right across the floor, but he was pushing with technique into my tension, and I did not have enough to make a break balance any more, and he did not pursue his push with his other skills. I am not saying that I am or was ever better than Mort, just that I became relaxed enough so that I could avoid that kind of push, which was what he was trying to teach me all along. Those too, were wonderful, magical days.

I learned just in time, as my now ex–wife was tired of spending any Sundays away from her parents and we were not to go back after that. It is a very good thing for my training and teaching that my breakthrough came just when it did.

Mort was and is a true friend. He wrote a wonderful book, *The Nine Dragons Saga*, a real page-turner. We exchange emails. He keeps me up to date, with pictures of the members of our T'ai Chi family that he has stayed in touch with.

Lou Kleinsmith – He pushed and we laughed

He was another of the senior six, the senior students of Professor Cheng in New York. He would catch my balance, and then bounce me left, bounce me right and then, perhaps, bounce me away (in a short push). Make no mistake, there were many who could push me, without having such skills, but because of his skills, Lou was the most fun to play with. He played with me, toyed with me really, like the game was sport aikido, in which he was dan ranked, as well. He would push me gently, off balancing me, and then when I started to go, he would catch my body, without permitting me to catch my balance, and push me again in another direction, perhaps at 90 degrees from the first push and then he would do it again, and again. Each a small push, a gentle push, each time pushing me just enough so that I could not regain my balance. In the end, he would let me fly and we would both laugh. I do not know why we laughed, but we did. There was a giddiness to it. His pushing skills were amazing, and what he did with them was qualitatively different from anyone else.

Stanley Israel - The more about Stan that I promised

With Stan there was a sense of his power, and not that light feel that Lou had. You were just powerfully, irresistibly, pushed away. Stanley would catch your center, or not, and then move you. It did not seem to matter if he had your center, you were gone either way. You knew you could not resist. Stanley was like a giant wave. Another thing about Stanley was his foothold, or rooting technique. He could root with no foot back. He was standing narrow and short, but you could not push him off his center. If you were determinedly attacking, he would roll his center a bit for you, so you could feel that he neutralized. He did not have to, but he did it, almost as if to say, that was a good push, I think I will acknowledge that, and then he would just forcefully bounce you away.

Professor said that Stanley had good push hands skill, and he never said that about anyone else that I am aware of. And Professor pushed a lot with Stanley, or should I say, pushed Stanley a lot, at the Association. Some of that is on film or video and may be seen. I pushed a lot with Stanley also, or rather was pushed a lot by Stanley, as my attempts to push him were quickly rooted or neutralized and counter pushed. We pushed most Saturdays after class from late 1967 to the end of 1969 in the back room at Midwood Judo Center, before I joined Professor's school. I decorated the walls from Stanley's power pushing, sometimes for hours at a time.

Lest you think Stanley was a natural, know that he had learned

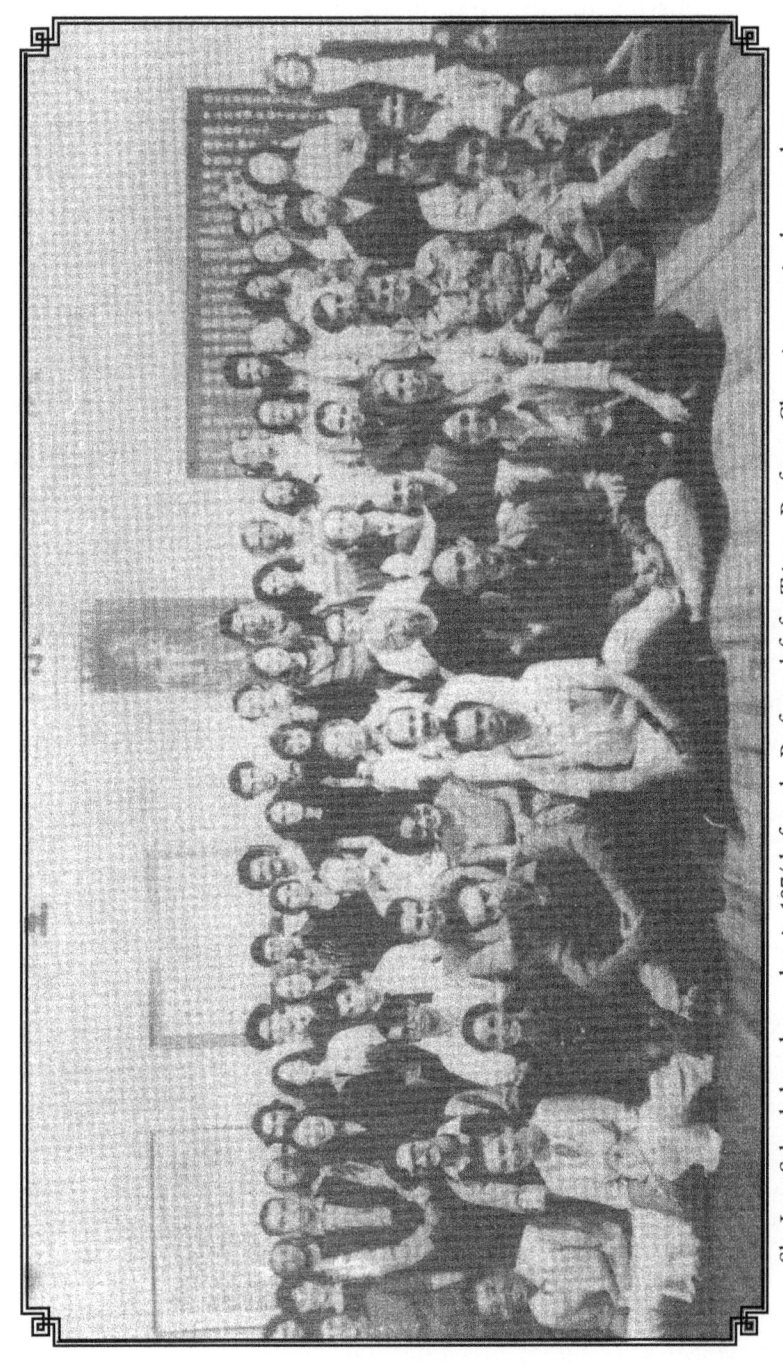

Shr Jung School class photo taken in 1974 before the Professor left for Taiwan. Professor Cheng is center in the second row. The author is seated four places to the left. The empty space at right is where photographer Ken Van Sickle had been sitting.
Photo credit: Kenneth Van Sickle.

IN THE PRESENCE OF CHENG MAN-CH'ING

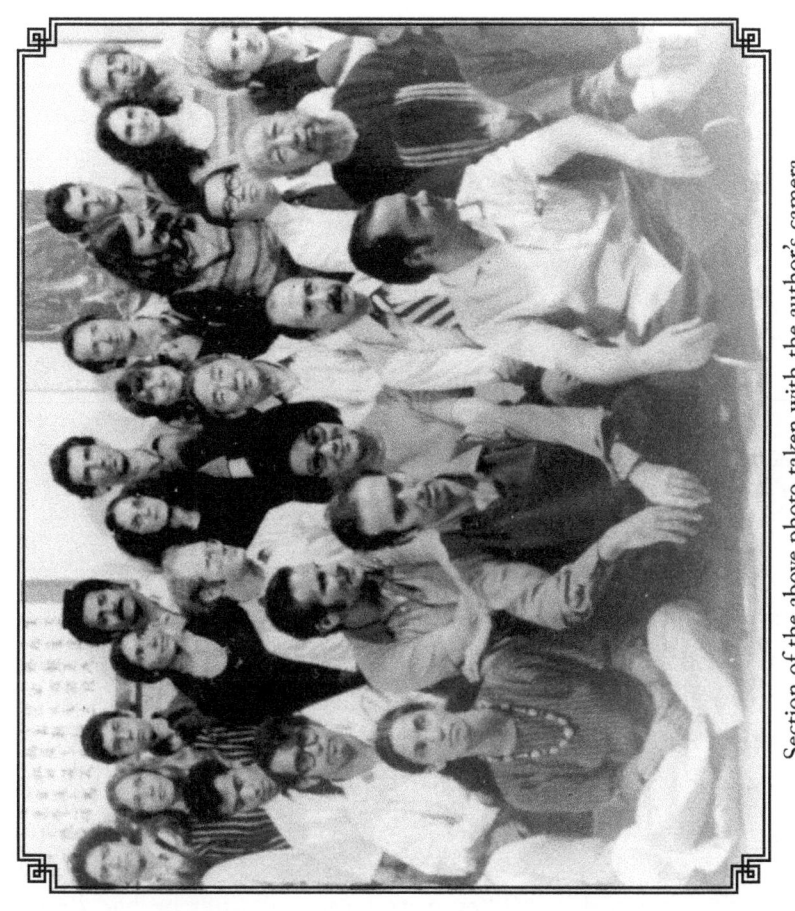

Section of the above photo taken with the author's camera.

Photo credit: Kenneth Van Sickle.

the hard way, like most of the rest of us. Stanley told me that when he was learning, he took heavy pushes from Professor till he would collapse right down on the floor. Eventually, he figured out that he had to try to neutralize the pushes. He could not just absorb, or take the push in, and push the pusher right back out, as he did with the pushes of just about everybody else. I do not know if he ever succeeded in neutralizing the Professor. I never saw him do it.

Tam Gibbs

Tam Gibbs was the senior student I knew the least well. I occasionally played sword dueling with him and often asked Professor questions and got Professor's medicine through him. Though I spoke with him about T'ai Chi, and had the rare casual conversation with him, he remained mostly a mystery to me. He was Professor's disciple and translator, along with Ed Young. They took turns translating at lectures and question and answer sessions, except for the formal lecture series at the Association, where Dr. Ren (of Columbia University) was the translator.

Ed Young

I met Ed Young when I joined the Association. Ed was one of Professor's translators along with Tam Gibbs. He was a senior student, quiet and somewhat reserved, but a nice guy, and unlike myself and some of the martial artists, a really gentle human being.

Around the time when Ed was teaching and I was assisting him at Yale (or some time shortly later), Ed gave me some rolled up sheets with art of his. They were copies of what he had drawn for a children's book. He had won a Caldecott Award for that art, and he was happy about it. I saved Ed's art and unfortunately hid it so well I cannot find it, if I did indeed manage to keep it through my divorce. It went missing when I had to move in a hurry. It was a time when many things went missing.

Maggie Newman

She is sweet and gentle of heart, but don't let that fool you. She is dedicated to self-perfection and serious, especially about T'ai Chi. She is a master teacher of Professor's form. When young, she was a kabuki dancer and also an aikido practitioner. In 1965 her picture was in Black Belt magazine doing aikido. I still have the issue with her picture in it.

Yet her T'ai Chi is wonderful to behold, and to be in her presence, and experience the exquisiteness of the peace that fills the room when she practices form, is just sublime. She is retired from teaching as of this writing, but she is still as sweet and wonderful as she ever was.

Herman Kauz

Herman was very protective of his friends and acquaintances. Once, as we were leaving the Association, at 211 Canal Street, when I was behind him going down the stairs and out the door, I slipped on some ice and yelped as I caught my balance. Herman turned in a fighting stance to see if I was in trouble. I was very happy that he seemed ready to defend me if necessary. While I thought I was pretty good in those days, I would have been happy to have his help, whether I needed it or not.

Not I nor anyone else I knew, except for the Professor, could get the best of Herman.

Another memory of the time at the Association, was that of his wife, a Hawaiian lady, bringing flowers to the Association and putting them on the table in the front room. I think she was arranging them. It is a fragment of a memory.

I told most of the rest of my Herman Kauz stories in the text above. I list him here because of his actions at the meeting of rebellious students. I felt that this made him, or should have made him, the seventh senior student. He had worked tirelessly for the school, and then he abruptly left. As I previously said, I do not know why.

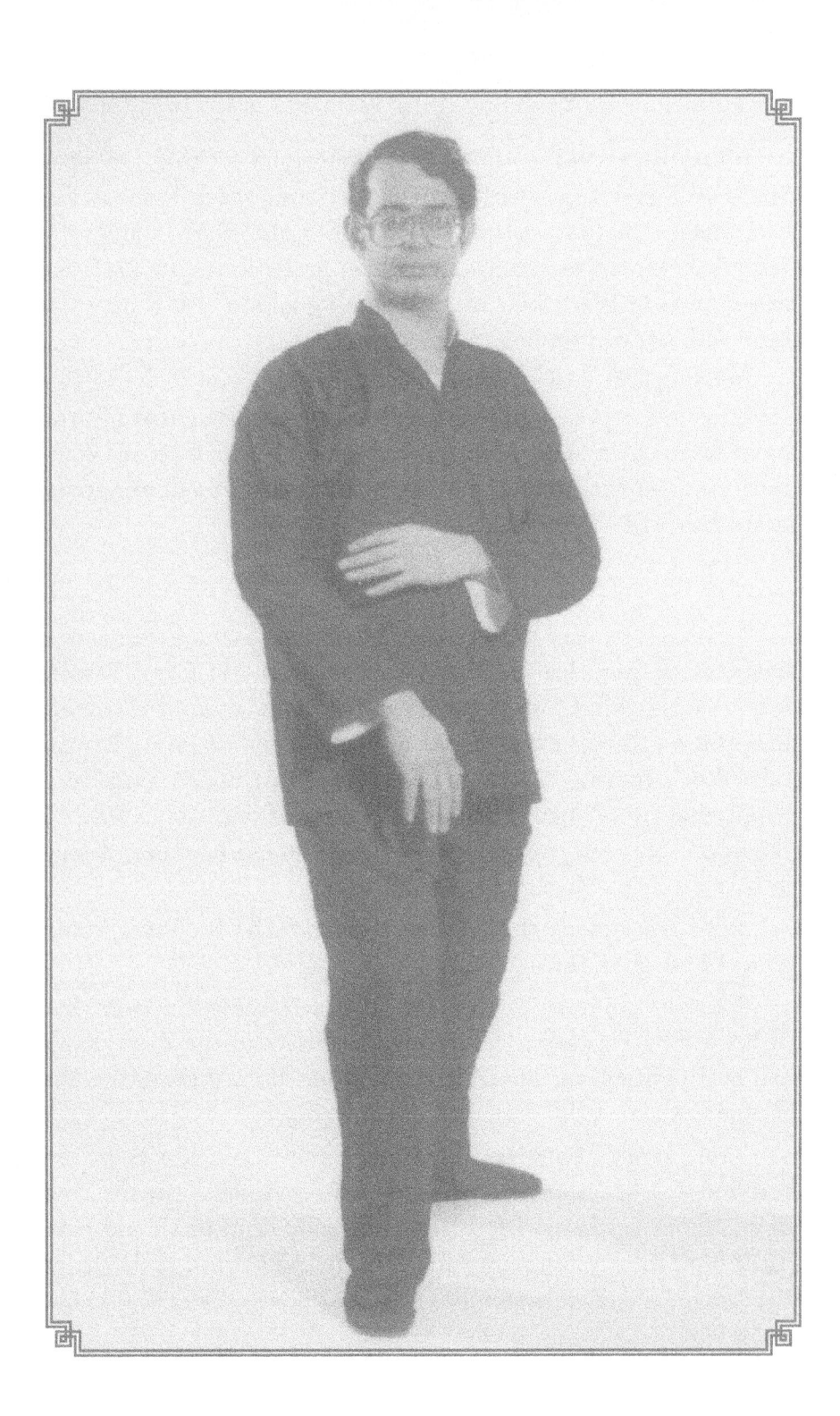

Chapter 10

Fellow Students

Kenneth Van Sickle

Kenneth was the official photographer. He had a lot more contact with professor than I did. I hope he gets out a book or memoir someday. It is by his permission that some of the pictures in this book are available. They are his. I am grateful for his kindness to me.

Lenny Antonucci

I knew Lenny Antonucci, from karate. He rented me space two nights a week in his martial arts school on 20th Avenue. This was another beginning for me, but that is another story, another school, another book. In the small world department, he is also a friend of Mario Napoli.

Harold Naiderman

Harold was an electrician. He was the Shr Jung's electrician, and he was much more than that. He was a protector of the Cheng family interests.

I do not know if he had any hand in the lawsuit, but I do know that he would tell anyone who was being disrespectful of the family to back off. I do not know if the Cheng family was aware of that.

When I needed to redo the electric lighting at my second martial arts school, at 4103 10th Avenue (which had been half of a funeral parlor), I hired Harold to put in some electrical "high hat" fixtures. Again, I assisted him by holding wiring for him and fetching stuff and handing him tools.

Jon Gaines

He did the carpentry for the Shr Jung. We became friends around that time, and I guess you could say that I apprenticed in woodwork a bit with him when I hired him to put kitchen cabinets in what was at that time my upstairs tenant's apartment in Langham Street. He took a straight piece of molding, soaked it in water, and somehow made it make an S curve as I watched and learned. He taught me about the nature of wood, and, I am proud to say, I helped.

He had an ashram in Hawaii when he passed away.

Shep Shepard

Shep was a friend from the Association. We played push hands and hung out a lot, he even came to my house to play. We played in my basement, among the books. He really wanted to improve and he would play anyone he could get his hands on. He played Ben Lo when he came to visit. I have a picture of that.

Since Shep passed away, I can add no more than my frail memory about him. He was a very good guy.

Lawrence Galante

Lawrence joined the Shr Jung as a senior student of one of Professor Cheng's Chinese students in NYC. We soon became friends as well. In addition to T'ai Chi, he is a gifted homeopathic practitioner. I found that out when I went to Lawrence's apartment to hang out. He gave me some homeopathic medicine, and it worked.

Many years later I taught his girlfriend Toni. When I was young I had the energy to spend all week at work, in Westinghouse Vocational and Technical High School, and then teach karate, ju jitsu, T'ai Chi, and children's self-defense. Then, on Friday nights, when I was not running a lecture series at Patience T'ai Chi, I would go to Middletown New York to teach Gus and Peg Carayas's T'ai Chi class (they rented an old railroad station). I taught the T'ai Chi in exchange for taking their stretching class and learning their weight training methods. Toni was in that T'ai Chi class. A group of us often went to dinner after, and then on Saturday morning I still went to my martial arts school and taught all day, from 10:00 AM to 3:30 PM, running children's birthday parties after.

Robert Morningstar

I knew Robert Morningstar at that time as well. I took ads with him for years after, in Free Spirit magazine. We split up the territory, and I think he got the best of it. He got Manhattan, where his school was, I got Brooklyn, where my school was, and my student Marc Isaacs got Long Island, where his school was. Forgive me Robert, I just do not remember any stories about hanging with you in the Shr Jung. Recently we met at a New Life Expo where he was speaking. (I was helping my friend, Gail Thackray and, when time permitted, hanging out with other friends, Jeff Gold, and Tim Bracci). He is a good acquaintance, and so I apologize here for not remembering more details. Perhaps if we get together we can bring some of our relationship back to my mind.

Wolfe Lowenthal

I played push hands with him at the Shr Jung. He has a wonderful ego, and remained soft and pliable no matter what. I pushed him with strength at first. Then I realized I could listen to him, follow him and catch him with sensitivity, and I pushed him with a lot less force.

My student, Jill Basso, wanted to attend his class. In very traditional old school style, he made her get written permission from me, to tell him that it was OK.

And Other People

I was acquainted with **Bataan and Jane Faigo** but they were just people I said hello and goodbye to, I did not really know them. I knew who **Carol Yamasaki** was, but did not know her any better than Bataan and Jane. She teaches T'ai Chi in Michigan, so I occasionally refer people to her. I did not know that **Katy Cheng** was another of Professor's daughters at that time either. I remember her as a very pretty, very attractive Chinese girl who was at the Shr Jung. She remembers me as someone who was constantly following after her father, either taking notes or using an audiocassette tape player, trying to learn everything I could. I knew **Frank Wong**, at the Shr Jung. I meet students of his wherever I go in the South East. I acquainted myself with **Judith Friedman** after the fact, as it was her child who is crying on my audiotape of one of Professor's talks. I am also occasionally in touch with **Phil Carter**, who was there, though I have no clear memory of us hanging out at the time. Sorry Phil. But we also became email friends.

Towards the end of my stay at the Shr Jung, I became friends with **Claire Hooten**. She got me into the Sheepshead Bay adult education program as a T'ai Chi teacher, and when they were taken over by Kingsborough Community College Division of Continuing

Education, I taught for them too. I taught T'ai Chi as well as self-defense for children and adults. Eventually I passed those classes on to students of mine. Finally, I taught a one-credit course in T'ai Chi for the Health and Physical Education Department of Kingsborough Community College from the fall of '87 to the spring of '95 as an adjunct instructor. I was laid off in spring of '95 in Governor Pataki's budget cuts. I resumed teaching at Kingsborough in the fall of 2010, and finally retired from it in December of 2015. I met many good friends as a result of Claire's kindness to me.

I met **Robert W. Smith** in 1975 at Professor's memorial service at the Shr Jung in New York and we took some pictures together. I was not in touch with him for quite some time after. I renewed our acquaintance in New York at William C. C. Chen's in the 1990s. He was giving a talk and showing some film. The only way to talk to him was to get on the autograph line, and so I did. I wanted to renew our acquaintance and give him copies of some of the pictures that we had taken in 1975. He autographed one of his pictures before he realized they were gifts. We got a laugh out of that. We got together later and we spoke of old times. He wanted me to have a copy of his newest book, and said to call the publisher for it. The publisher was not so cooperative. Long story short, I had to buy it on Amazon.com.

We kept in touch by phone until he passed. He was a delightful conversationalist, always full of the latest T'ai Chi news and gossip.

Apologies

I spent time with a lot of people at the Association and at the Shr Jung, so if I left you out, I apologize. My memory has faded some, and that is part of why I write, to establish a record so that it will not all be forgotten. I also write to share my experiences of a magical time in my life. So if I did not mention you and we were friends in those times, please call and remind me. Let's chew the fat about times gone by, and you may be in the next edition of this book, if I get so lucky to have one.

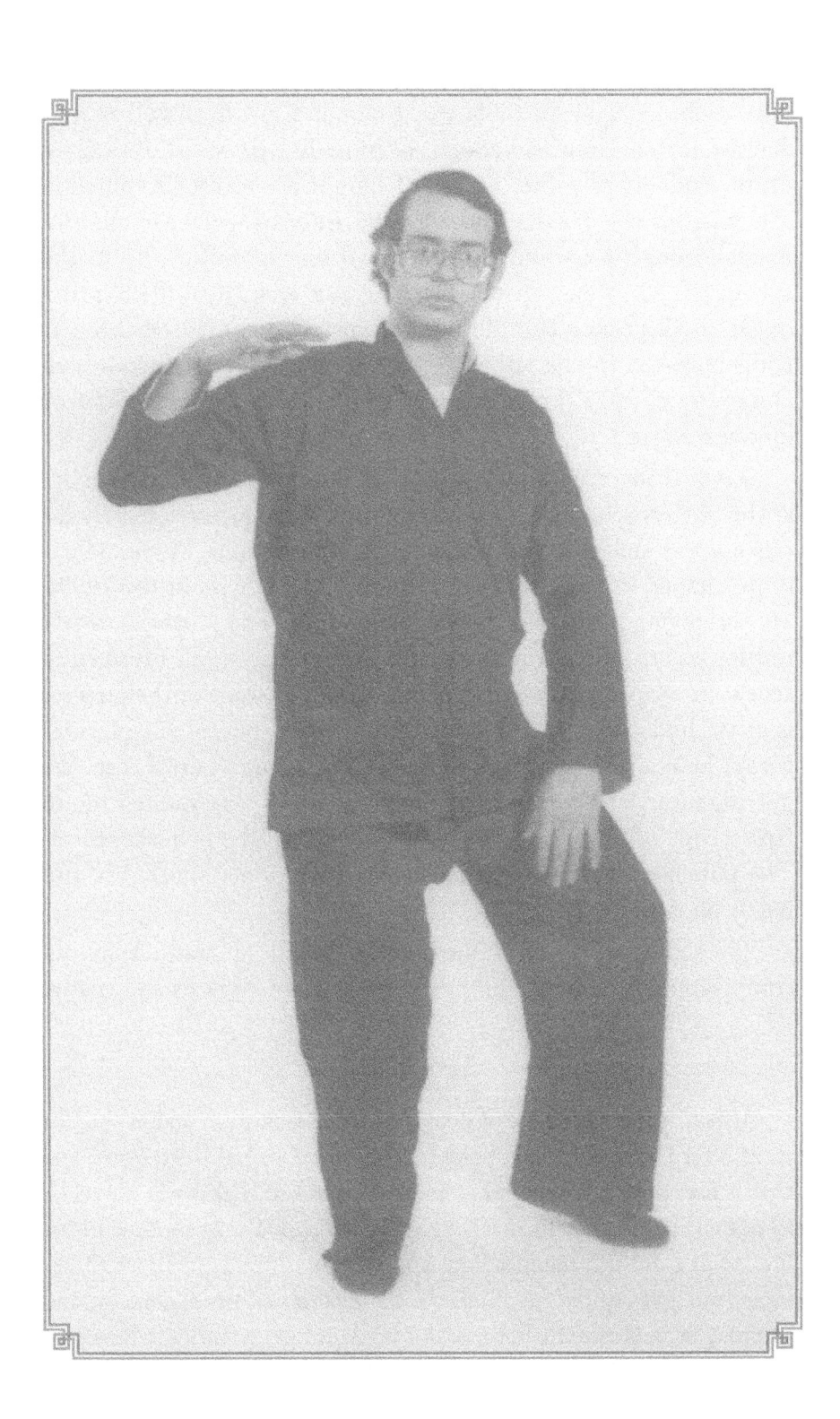

Chapter 11

The Professor's Wisdom, Teachings and Habits

Professor told us he had studied seven years with Yang Cheng Fu. He said he had a private class from 5:00 AM to 6:00 AM and then went to classes during the day and also helped Master Yang to teach those classes. Studying with Yang Cheng Fu was kind of a full time occupation for Professor. But when he wanted to teach T'ai Chi on his own, Professor shortened what he was taught, with Yang Cheng Fu's permission, so as to get to what he considered to be the essence of T'ai Chi. He needed to do this originally to teach the troops, as he was T'ai Chi teacher in Chung King for Chaing Kai Shek's nationalist army fighting the Japanese.

In fact, there was a story we were told of Professor taking a challenge from a British boxer in Chung King. He avoided, blocked, and parried the Englishman and then pushed him off the raised platform they were sparring on.

Professor kept refining those skills, and he could see the martial in everything he taught. But in each generation he taught a version that was becoming less overtly martial and seemingly more energetic, and more about health.

You also should know that Professor had healed himself of tuberculosis with T'ai Chi. A Master of Chinese medicine, he had full command of the health benefits as well.

So while he was getting to the essence of T'ai Chi with a shorter form, I believe he was also refining what that essence should be over his years of practice and teaching. This is just my opinion, after having studied Professor's short form with Stan Israel (3 years), with Professor Cheng (5 years) and Yang Family Long Form with Zhang Lu-Ping (10 years). Master Zhang learned Yang family long form from Fu Zhong Wen. As a result, I have some insights as to where the form came from, as well as where it was going.

The unvarnished truth

With knowledge comes understanding and with understanding comes wisdom. While I give my understanding (interpretations) of what Professor said, I wish to do my best to give the unvarnished teachings of my Master, so that you can go over his words as exactly as I have, and do. Though Katy Cheng says that he is not well interpreted or well translated, at least you can have as much information as I. I have given my interpretations so you can have the benefit of my thoughts and explanations, varnishings, if you will, of Professor's wisdom.

One of Professor's students from Taiwan who came here said that in Taiwan they were envious of the access to him that we had, and the instruction that we got from Professor. He indicated that they rarely got to see him do even a complete round of form. I guess, if that is so, that he realized that if he wanted to teach us Westerners, the traditional Chinese way, demonstrating and letting the student pick it up, was not going to work. I, for one, am grateful. I could never have learned it that way.

Practice: Day and Night

Professor Cheng said that you should do T'ai Chi as soon as you wake up in the morning.

I have to brush my teeth first and use the bathroom, and so it is the third thing I do in the morning.

Professor Cheng said that T'ai Chi should be the last thing you do before bed.

This I do. But when I get to bed I often watch TV, so maybe I do not do this as well as I should either.

Professor Cheng used to tell us to practice every morning and every evening, every day of our lives. In sickness and in health.

This I do.

Professor thought T'ai Chi should bracket sleep. He took this very seriously. He used to say, if we had to give up some breakfast, do it and practice. If we had to give up some sleep, do it and practice. Practicing every day, morning and night, is an important discipline, and will bear the fruit of the benefits of T'ai Chi. How unimportant is losing a little breakfast or sleep, compared to getting the benefits of T'ai Chi?

Commentary

There are some things I have discovered about doing this:

In the event that you are doing this and you are more awake before doing the morning round, instead of after, examine yourself. Did you sleep badly? Did you wake up tense? If the answer to either is yes, that is the reason: T'ai Chi relaxes you. So if you wake up tense, and thereby awake, naturally it will relax you. When it does, your sleepiness will begin to come out. Sleeping well becomes important to the practice T'ai Chi.

If you practice at night and you are less sleepy after than you were before, then the T'ai Chi is waking you up. In that case you probably had a tense day, but not a physically demanding day and your body is being awakened by the T'ai Chi. T'ai Chi relaxes, so if your body is tense, your practice will relax you and leave you alert, and calm. If your body is tired it will make you sleepy.

If you have had a good day, and a good sleep, you will be awake in the morning and sleepy at night.

Always keep moving when you practice T'ai Chi.

Professor said to always move as you practice. Do not pause. Do not stop, from beginning to end. Do the T'ai Chi as one movement, one piece. I asked him if we stopped when we were about to reverse our direction. He said no, it's all one move. Do not stop, do not pause.

Like the Silk Worm

Further, he went on to say in talks with us that we should move at one constant speed for a round of form. He gave the example of a silkworm making silk. It moves at one pace. If it speeds up, the silk thread becomes thinner. If it slows down the silk thread becomes thicker. If the silkworm stops, and then starts again the thread breaks. But if it continues to move at one speed, the strand of silk is perfectly uniform throughout.

Chi Moves Too

He also said to keep the ch'i moving through out each round of form. It does not stop from beginning to end.

Space for T'ai Chi

Professor Cheng, used to say that we should be able to do the T'ai Chi in a four-foot by four-foot area.

Commentary

I have found that, with the correction step I used to take, I used a corridor, of around six by three feet, though with additional correction steps I guess four by three feet would do. I found I needed the width in the footage because to do the posture, snake creeps up (squatting single whip), you need to reach out, otherwise I would think it could be done in a three- by two-foot space. Now that I have a nice apartment, I have allotted half a room to T'ai Chi practice, and I do not worry about space any more.

Some people have supposed that like karate kata, you should start and finish in the same place (The Japanese martial arts call this embusen). I have not found that to be the case, without correction steps. I can end up in the same place, east to west. However, if I take proper stances, I am further south at the close of the form.

Spit as Medicine

Professor said, when you first wake up, if you do not rush off to brush your teeth, you can take that first saliva in your mouth and use it as a rubbing medicine.

Professor's Massages

Kidney: His kidney massage for health involved doing forty-nine repetitions with both wrists lightly against the kidneys, pushing the wrists down towards the floor. You keep your weight on one foot. Then you do another forty-nine with your weight on the other foot. He recommended that it be done between 5:00 PM and 7:00 PM for best effect.

Stomach: You do sixty-four with each hand for the stomach/abdomen. You make a fist and circle it lightly around the stomach. Going across the top of the circle, it is palm down, thumb knuckle against your stomach. Going across the bottom, it is palm up, pinky knuckle against your abdomen. You do this one hand at a time. It should be done after eating, especially after a heavy meal.

Eyes: You do thirty-six repetitions with both hands at

the same time, one on each socket. You use the thumb bottom knuckle. Go from the side of the head, with both hands, on the outside of the eye, but inside the socket, under it and then up, coming back to the outside just under the eyebrows. Important, keep your hands and knuckles out of your eyes, and do it gently.

Lost Massage: I have notes about a chest massage, but no memory or description. My notes say 21 times lightly down in the chest on each side.

Health

Professor said if you have good health, do not take it for granted, for that is the beginning of bad health.

Directions, Northern Exposure

Professor said you should face north when you practice T'ai Chi in this hemisphere, and south in the southern hemisphere. He also said you should sleep with your head facing north, or east if you cannot do north, to be more alert. If you practice, or sleep, facing south or west, it will make you more sleepy, and less alert. Again, this is in the northern hemisphere; in the southern, the opposite applies.

Breathing to the Tan T'ien

Professor Cheng used to tell us to find and breathe to our tan t'iens and focus our ch'i there. By doing so, we inhale the ch'i (energy) of heaven (the atmosphere), mixed with the ch'i of earth, and bring it to our own internal energy storage point: the tan t'ien (a kind of internal battery). There it mixes with the energy of your blood in your body. This was not just instruction for doing T'ai Chi, but for doing everything, walking, talking, eating, everything. Always breath to your tan t'ien.

COMMENTARY

You can feel it, when you breathe to the tan t'ien. At first you think it is your breath that you are feeling, because it feels like breath. But you do not have any lungs going straight down your chest and abdomen to a spot under your navel, so you eventually realize that it is the ch'i, or energy that you are experiencing as breath.

MORE ON THE TAN T'IEN

Professor said that you should breathe to your tan t'ien as much as possible, and that your breathing should be as quiet as you can get it.

COMMENTARY

As with many things I was taught, I have some comments about breathing to the tan t'ien based on my years of practice.

First, a suggestion on how to help you to find it, for those of you who are having trouble:

Place your pointer and middle fingers of the right hand about an inch under your navel and breathe.

If these fingers of the right hand won't attract the ch'i,

Try the pinky and ring fingers of the left hand.

One set of fingers should work. Either the first two fingers of the right (the most yang fingers of the yang hand), or last two fingers of the left (the most yin fingers of the yin hand), have the best chance of working.

To which I will add, as you breathe all day long; as you walk, or work, or eat, or play, you can feel your tan t'ien. You can do this whether you are practicing T'ai Chi or not. When the tan t'ien is full, you should stop (just my opinion). I have had the ch'i flash back from my tan t'ien up to my heart/chest area. You may feel this as an explosion of heat in the chest. Also, if you do it too much the opposite may appear to happen. You may feel low on energy as your tan t'ien absorbs all your energy. At other times you may feel a bubbling on the head as you breathe to your tan t'ien, this is the energy spontaneously flowing in the microcosmic orbit. If these things are happening, take some time off from breathing to your tan t'ien, as much time as you find helpful, from a couple of hours to a couple of days.

When you store enough energy in your tan t'ien, it will flow to your fingers and later to your feet as you practice. This is the macrocosmic orbit. You do not have to do anything for this to happen, but it is helpful to do the proper inhales and exhales of the form along with the postures. It is kind of like T'ai Chi is CPR of energy, and the ch'i will flow to your fingers and then to your bubbling wells (more on that later).

Nosy

Professor Cheng invited me to put my fingers under his nose and hold them there for a couple of minutes. He would talk and obviously needed to inhale and exhale. He was not holding his breath, he was alive and breathing, presumably to his tan t'ien. And yet his breath was too quiet to feel, whatever else it was.

He advocated breathing, inhaling and exhaling, through the nose, with your tongue on the hard palate, the roof of the mouth. He also advocated practicing breathing until you were able to do a 30 second inhale and a 30 second exhale with no discomfort. At this point I am up to 20 to 25 seconds, but I am still working on it.

How to breathe
(You are alive, so you thought you knew, right?)

Professor Cheng gave us specific instructions on how to breathe during the practice of the form. He told us to inhale on yang movements and exhale on yin movements. This is the opposite of karate breathing. This method is not well understood today, and it has become controversial.

Professor Cheng gave us two different reasons at different times. One reason for the inhale and another for the exhale. Please remember for this explanation T'ai Chi Ch'uan has been called swimming in air.

Inhale: A fish swims in water. The fish is not aware of the weight of the mass of the water as we experience it from outside the water when we put our hands into the water. We, living in the air, are very aware of the mass of the water.

On the other hand, we live in a substance called the air, which also has mass. We are not aware of the mass of the air, as the fish is not aware of the mass of the water. When we inhale on a punch, we add to our mass and so to the momentum of our punch. We are making our strikes heavier.

COMMENTARY

I might add that if you drive at, say fifty or sixty miles an hour and stick your hand out the window, you will get an idea of what mass he is talking about, as you feel the resistance/heaviness of the air.

For the martial artists among our readers, when you throw an exhaled punch, it is like an iron bar, shot as a missile. It cannot easily change directions, or adjust to a changing situation. An inhaled punch leaves you in control, because you are more alive, less focused so you can change directions or collapse against a block or changing the punch to an elbow strike if the block is low on your forearm, near the hand.

Another time the Professor said that it is foolish to inhale on a contracting move, because we are taking away our internal space when we do that. To see this, turn your waist to one side, while inhaling. Then do the same move while exhaling. How much more internal space will you have for the turn? How much farther will you be able to turn by exhaling on contracting moves? By exhaling we are getting out of our own way.

When neutralizing, it is always helpful to have more internal room.

Professor said the breath should be long, quiet, slow, smooth, relaxed, and comfortable. He also said a good breath should be a comfortable thirty second inhale and a comfortable thirty second exhale. He explained that the inhales and exhales of the form conform to the yin and yang of the movements, and were, therefore, irregular, conforming to the postures. He also said we should never be fully inhaled or fully exhaled throughout the form.

He went on to say that you should never be more than thirty-five percent exhaled during any posture of the T'ai Chi form, and you should breathe silently.

In other applications of the breathing, he said a good time to attack was at the point of the change of breath, as in when a person is fully inhaled and about to exhale or fully exhaled, and about to inhale. At that time the person was most vulnerable. The most dangerous time to attack was when the opponent is in the middle of his exhale.

Ch'i of Heaven: City and Country

Professor said the ch'i in the city is not as good as the ch'i in the country. I do not recall that he ever explained what "good" is. But, he said that some people have trouble benefiting from the country ch'i because it is too strong for them and they cannot cope with it.

Bubbling Well

Professor Cheng said that the bubbling well (kidney 1, for the acupuncturists among us) is a hollow point with no muscle in it. When you can flatten it and get it on the ground it makes a great point around which to organize your balance. Also, our ch'i, or energy, can be made to go there. Professor said that once we find our bubbling well, we should breathe to it and feel the ch'i we bring there at all times. He said we could find the bubbling well and bring ch'i there in our T'ai Chi practice. Once found, we should always feel it, and be aware of it with every step we take, even when just standing around.

He said we should focus our balance around it. That at first we might need the whole foot to balance, but eventually, as we focus on the bubbling well, we would need less space on our foot to balance.

COMMENTARY

As we work on finding and using our bubbling well, our balance might shift to the front or back half of the foot, then to a silver dollar sized area around the bubbling well. Then, when lost, we need not fall. Instead we can just wobble on our foot. Eventually we can organize our balance onto a smaller sized area on the front of the foot, and then to an area that can be represented by ever smaller coins, until eventually, in theory, you could balance on the area of a compass point in the center of your bubbling well.

SHOES

Professor said we should wear leather- or cloth-soled shoes to feel the ch'i (electromagnetic force) of the earth. Rubber soles, he said, would insulate us from the ch'i of the earth.

COMMENTARY

But rubber soles are so much more comfortable, and so I mostly wear the comfortable shoes.

MEDITATION

When asked if he practiced seated meditation separately from T'ai Chi, Professor said, "No, I practice T'ai Chi and it is enough, it is complete."

When he was asked if he did ch'i kung separately from T'ai Chi, and he again said "I do T'ai Chi" to answer the question.

COMMENTARY

So T'ai Chi was his meditation and his ch'i kung, as well as his martial art and his health practice.

No sweat

I know this is counter-intuitive, but Professor did not want us to sweat in our practice. This was important enough to him that he gave those of us who were there at the time a talk about this. Professor Cheng used to tell us, if we sweat, to stop practice, as we are losing our ch'i.

COMMENTARY

As a young man strengthening my legs I had some sweating to do, and I did not understand. As a beginner, you must sweat as you strengthen and learn. So, while in the sweating stage, I wrote this instruction down for future reference. Today I do understand. I do not necessarily follow it, but I do understand. If you can control your exertion, contain your heat and bodily fluids, you can develop your ch'i in a much more efficient way. Still, this is often easier said than done. I would guess that you have to be at a level beyond mine to put this into regular practice. If I ever get there I will let you know. In the meantime, I still need to strengthen my legs, so I am still sweating.

I do have a cheat for this: When I sweat, I wet my T-shirt with perspiration. At that point, a breeze, any breeze, will cool and dry me.

Ch'i exercise notes

In one of our conversations, as I have mentioned previously, Professor suggested that I do raise hands back and down for at least one hour a day. I came to call it the ch'i exercise because of what it did for my hands and feet. I felt a lot of ch'i as I did the exercise with the proper inhales and exhales. After about six months I stopped, as I thought I pretty much had what Professor was aiming at. It served me well, so I thought I would pass it on.

You should begin the "ch'i exercise" as if you are a blow up doll and the air nozzle is in your spine behind your shoulders. As it fills your arms, they rise. When pressure is sufficient, it breaks the seals at your wrists and your hands fill and rise to become just parallel with the ground. As that happens, your elbows drop a bit, straight down with most people. Then you remove the air hose and your arms deflate. As they do, your hands fall over (fingers point forty-five degrees or so down as they just hang there), and your wrists come back to your shoulders as your elbows bend. At this point in the exercise, that image is finished.

Next image: Your arms become as Chinese scales and you rebalance them as you straighten your hands so a straight line exists from the tops of your fingernails to the inside of the elbow pit. I call this reattaching your hands. As you change the position of your hands, the elbows fall back slightly in this rebalance. But it is not enough just to move those elbows back, you have to feel where the elbows want to adjust to on the fulcrum of your shoulders.

Last image: your hands are parachutes, filling with air. They float gently down, as the elbow joints open.

More is less

Professor said that you can't benefit from over practice. It is like the stars in the sky, they only move so far in a day, a predetermined amount of movement as you watch the sky. This is an analogy to how much we can improve in one day's practice. You can practice too little and not get the all the benefit of a day's practice, but practicing too much will not help you get more benefit than you can get in a day. Only so much can be done in a day, more practice on the same day is redundant and not helpful. So he urged us to do it right, rather than more often. He did not believe that we could improve by more practice in a day, but believed we should practice more days instead. That is one of the principles of T'ai Chi. Practice all the days of your life.

COMMENTARY

This was another piece of advice I did not take at the time. As a youngster, I was full of energy and wanted to practice a lot in order get "the secrets." Now that I have practiced many more days, many more years, I see the wisdom of this. Every day has its own obstacles to practice, its own challenges. Succeed every day and you will benefit. Every day of my life is practice. I recommend it.

MONEY, MONEY, MONEY, MONEY ...

Professor Cheng used to tell us that he wanted us to be paid for teaching. He told us that T'ai Chi is a valuable skill that we have taken time and effort to learn. He thought we should be paid for the effort we put in to learn T'ai Chi, as well as for passing on this valuable skill. He also said that people often do not appreciate what does not cost them something.

COMMENTARY

Once you are teaching, you need to decide if you will charge for the lessons you give. Many in CMC (Cheng Man-Ch'ing) T'ai Chi do not charge for it, and that is their choice. You who are teachers have been given this gift. It is up to you to decide how you will share it.

FOOD RULES

As mentioned in Chapter 7, Professor said he ate congee (rice cooked until it is watery), in the morning, green vegetables and rice with peanuts at noon and rice, or more congee, in the evening. He said that you should eat the big meal mid-day. He also said he had a little brandy on cold mornings, as it helped him get his ch'i flowing.

He said that man is like the sun, weak in the morning and

the evening. He said that we did not appreciate the amount of energy it takes to digest our food. It takes a lot, so we should eat accordingly.

He advocated eating breakfast at 6:00 AM, lunch at noon, and dinner at 6:00 PM.

He said, without explanation, that we should eat as little meat as possible. He said something else about food, and I do not understand it to this day: During the evening meal we should absorb the tastes of the food. (I think without taking in too much food?)

More food rules

Within an hour of your practice:

Professor said not to eat an hour before or after practice.

When I was working it was not possible to take this advice.

The Seventy Percent rule

Professor said to eat only until you are seventy percent full. Then wait fifteen minutes to half an hour and see how you feel. If you are content in your stomach, you are finished with that meal.

When I was working, and even now, when I am eating in a restaurant, it is not an easy thing to do. But at home I try to do this.

Even more food rules, and less popular ones, too

Professor Cheng said that drinking cold was like diving into a cold lake. They body likes hot drinks because they are closer to body temperature. The body feels shock when we drink cold. So, as we would not plunge our outsides into ice water, we should not plunge our insides into it.

Commentary

I cannot stand ice-cold water on my body. But as of this writing, I like a cold drink, preferably on the rocks. So I hope my body can continue to tolerate the internal freezing that often passes as a good cold drink.

Eating bitter, it's not what you think

Professor said we should eat bitter. This was not about diet, but about practice: training the legs.

It was said of Professor Cheng that he trained so hard that he could not climb into bed at night, so tired were his legs.

Commentary

My analogous situation was that I had to hold on to the banisters, going down the stairs at 87 Bowery, after class, so tired were my legs in spite of my previous judo, karate, ju jitsu, and running.

Back to bitter

Professor told us that our legs are the peasants, and need to be worked hard. You need to go home exhausted and with spent legs while you are learning. This was something that Professor said a lot. He had very strong legs. Mario Napoli remembers having been told, by Stanley, that he was invited to feel Professor's legs, and they were as hard as rocks.

Commentary

Yet he also said, do not sweat in your practice, you will lose your ch'i. From this I deduced, though he did not say it, as a student, exhaust your legs, sweat as much as you need to in order to make your legs strong. Then, when you are low and deep, do it effortlessly, focusing on the breath, the ch'i etc.

The fruits of the bitter tree

When our legs got strong, he wanted us to move in a relaxed way, with the proper breathing, in perfect body alignment, elbows and knees, wrists and ankles, shoulders and hips, with the spine straight, moving, gliding, as one unit.

COMMENTARY

The one time that a group of Chinese masters really enthusiastically approved of the form I was doing, I was doing a really low and slow, effortless version of Professor Cheng's form. They were so happy with it they invited me to dinner. My legs were as strong then as they have ever been. You really need to work hard to keep strong legs, as the strength will leak out as you age if you do not practice really vigorously, regularly.

On Standing to Strengthen the Legs

This is a complex question, believe it or not. This is because on the one hand, Professor placed no emphasis on standing meditation, tree hugging etc., but that is not the whole story.

He advocated that we hold static postures for lengths of time.

He shared with us two postures that would be good for our leg strength if we held them. He described how to stand in those postures for maximum leg benefit. He recommended Single Whip and Raise Hands, or Play Guitar to strengthen the legs. In Play Guitar, for example, he said to imagine the more outstretched hand as being heavy and pulling you down into your root.

While he never told us to hold static postures in class, to be in his class was to hold many postures for long lengths of time as he was correcting people, and he took his time correcting people. We got to stand in many postures in his class, for fifteen to twenty minutes at a time, including Golden Cock and Heel Kick, on one foot. As I have stated before, when I got to the stairs after class, I had to hold on to the banister to go down, my legs were so tired. With my cross country and martial arts background, my legs were stronger than most people's legs, but not strong enough for his correction class.

Once You Have Tasted Bitter and Learned

Things to concentrate on: Once you have learned the form and strengthened the legs, then you are ready to learn the form again, at a more advanced level. T'ai Chi form is in the feelings: Professor said breathe to the tan t'ien and feel your breath. It should be very quiet, long or short as the posture requires, done at a slow rate. It should be smooth and relaxed.

Feel the straightness of the spine, the ch'i in the fingers, and the bubbling well of the hands (not the heart point) and feet. Feel the turning of the hips, and the placement of the feet, then what you are walking on as well. Feel the placement of the knees and elbows, and their alignment. There are many things to feel, and these are just a few.

Other Things From My Notes

- Relax.
- Feel the head as if suspended from above.
- Feel the tail as if with a lead weight on it, being pulled down below.
- Feel your legs.
- Feel your fingers.
- Keep the fingers evenly spaced (if you can).
- When the ch'i is relaxed, the head will be clear.
- Keep cool.
- Your head should feel like it is floating.
- Ch'i to the tan t'ien.
- Keep your head at the same level as you move forward or backwards as you practice.
- A bobbing head as the weight shifts from foot to foot is not correct.
- You should sit back and come forward with your head on the same level as an exercise until you have it correct.
- Only turn to the side a moderate amount during push hands, but turn fully/completely during exercises and practice.

- Work to expand your flexibility when you are exercising, by going to the corners. But when playing push hands, you should always have a little extra flexibility.
- In the form, one side of the body is always yin and the other side yang.
- When asked about the raise hands back and down, he explained that the yin/yang split was across the waist. The body is divided top from bottom.
- The most important part of the T'ai Chi form is the beginning.
- T'ai Chi is a unique exercise because you move your ch'i and your organs. When the form is finished, the organs settle.
- He said he does not talk too much for fear of losing his ch'i. But that we have so little ch'i it does not matter. He was asked if this use of ch'i meant breath. He said no, that it was his tan t'ien or abdomen ch'i. We must always use it to operate, to function.
- The bones are hollow, like noodles, so that blood, or ch'i can flow through them.
- Single whip's health benefit is for the lungs. The farther back you can hold your right arm, the better it is for the lungs.
- He also said that you can negate the health benefit of that posture by doing it on the other side.
- T'ai Chi is done as it is for a reason. Doing a round on the other side negates the health benefits.

The eyes

He said different things at different times about the eyes:
Keep them focused inward to the balance point on the head.
Keep your eyes relaxed and focused, as if on an opponent in push hands, as well as on your environment, during the form.

Be aware, and do not let the T'ai Chi form do you. You do the form. You become aware of your environment when you do the form.

COMMENTARY

I think he may have been alluding to a meditative round of form in the first direction, and in general form practice for the second and third, as he said these things at different times, in different contexts.

FURTHER COMMENT WITH AN EYE TO SELF-DEFENSE

It is just my opinion, but this second statement, as I have it in my notes, is as close as he ever got to the popular misconception that you should imagine an opponent in front of you when you do the form. He never said that in my hearing, he just said to be aware of what is in front of you, whether it is a person or a thing. There is a difference between seeing and imagining. Imagining is making patterns and making patterns takes away options, giving your opponent an advantage.

If you do this, imagining an opponent in front of you, it may be harder to face a real opponent should the occasion arise. This is because you are training your mind to be imagining what your visualized partner is doing. If you have imagined your imaginary opponent doing something that your actual opponent does not do, what happens then?

It is my thought, that you should approach any situation with no preconception, and go with the flow of your opponent. Let him give you the information you need and the momentum or stiffness you need to defeat him.

As a friend, Sensei Thomas Casale is fond of saying, "Practice does not make perfect, practice makes permanent." To which I add, if you have a higher goal, a picture of perfection that you are working to achieve, you can achieve it through practice. But if you think you are doing it perfectly, you will just keep on doing what you have been doing, and not improve.

T'ai Chi is about a lifetime of improvement, not a lifetime of being at whatever level you may find yourself when you think you have gotten it.

T'ai Chi form is multifaceted. Focus too soon or too hard on any one thing and you may lose the others.

This is particularly true of the martial applications in T'ai Chi, because the postures are multipurpose. One man's martial applications are not another's. So much depends on the individual. Many things will work. Another is that just seeing an opponent does not give you all the information you need. You need more: Where is his weight? What is his intention? These are just two that come immediately to my mind.

Doing the T'ai Chi

Do not let the T'ai Chi form do you. You do the form.

Musical commentary

You can see this most easily in the beginner's use of music in the practice of the form. He/she gets lost in the music and finds that he/she somehow has arrived at the end of their form. You need to stay alert in practice, and be more aware, not less, of what you are doing and seeing. Aware of your environs. To me, this use of music is not correct. Music can be used when you have achieved a certain amount of advancement. Use it by ignoring it and continuing as you would have done without it.

Sex, nope, not the good part you think you have been

WILLIAM C. PHILLIPS

WAITING FOR

Men

Professor had some pretty strong ideas on sexual abstinence. Or at least, moderation that seems like abstinence. Professor told us that we needed to regulate our sex lives. He said that if we did not, our ch'i would be expended, and our legs would become weak. He said we would walk stoop shouldered and be shorter than we had been when we got to our old age.

He said he was not advocating abstinence, but just self-regulation, and to be moderate with our orgasms. He also said this advice was for men, who use ch'i and valuable proteins in each ejaculation. He said the body draws these proteins from our legs.

He said the body draws out the best of us, our best proteins and our best energy (ch'i) to put in our semen and our orgasms, because a function of sex is to create the next generation.

And that the body uses the best stuff to create that next generation.

This was his regimen:

Between the ages of 16 to 24, we should indulge not more than once a week.

Between the ages of 24 to 32, once in two weeks.

Between the ages of 32 and 40 once in four weeks.

Between the ages of 40 and 48, once in eight weeks.

Between the ages of 48 and 56, once in sixteen weeks.

Between the ages of 56 and 64, once in thirty-two weeks.

Commentary

I never heard him go beyond that, so I do not know what he intended. It could be that if you are still alive, it does not matter after that. It also could be that maybe you did not have to wait more than 32 weeks, or, if you did, you might just forget what you were waiting for.

He would sometimes point out an old man walking hunched over with a cane and say that the man had had too much sex. He also said your legs would go if you had too much sex.

He said that this was because the semen had first call on the protein and nerve cells needed to create new life. So if we had too much sex, our semen would repeatedly be replenished with the stuff it needed to make new life, which was the same stuff we most needed to keep in our bodies in order to live a long and healthy life.

WOMEN

He said that women were different and could have more sex than men because they do not lose valuable proteins when they have an orgasm. He also said that women could burn out their blood ch'i if they indulged too often.

BOTH SEXES

The attitude you have during sexual intercourse is important, and can make a very big difference to the quality of sex you are having and to the quality of the experience of your sex partner.

If it is just about lust or even emotional love, it will burn out. But if each is concerned with the health and well-being of the other person, good sex can last a long time. (It will not become ordinary over the years). Also, with the right intention, it will be a healing, balancing experience. (Without right intention, it will be a tiring experience, especially for men.) The comments in parentheses are mine.

COMMENTARY

It is possible to not need sex, and to be relaxed through the practice of T'ai Chi. However, if you are developing tension, it is a quick release. You know it is not too much as long as you do not feel tired after. You should feel refreshed after sex, if you have released excess tension.

Bony ch'i

Professor said as part of the process of breathing and ch'i, you breathe to the tan t'ien. As you fill the tan t'ien, if you are sexually moderate, there will be an overflow of ch'i that will migrate to the marrow of the bones, and the bones will become essentially hard.

Professor on Push Hands

Professor said to root like a mountain. When you push, release your power like a tidal wave, or tornado. Be as sensitive as the air, like a quiet wind. Neutralize like a shadow.

Push through your sensitivity, and then comes your power. Another time he said almost the same thing, but perhaps a bit easier to understand. He said, "Push through your sensitivity and then when you feel it, connect to your power." (Feel the person's center being unbalanced, is my take on what "it" is.)

Swords

Professor said that your sword should be measured to you if you are buying a sword. It should measure from your tan t'ien to the floor, and it should feel light in your hand.

When I was taught sword form, I was taught it twice. First the movements and postures. When that was learned, then came the principles. Push the sword and follow it, use your hips to move the sword throughout the form. Lou Kliensmith drilled us in this.

(The first round of sword form is taught relatively slowly. The second at the speed of your sword, falling or being pushed. It has varying speeds.)

There were sword exercises that Professor wanted us to do to get control over the sword. He gave us one exercise in which we made loops with the sword. It is intended to help you to become softer and have greater control of the tip of the sword. The idea of it was that the handle makes a wide loop, as if it is rotating around a porthole, while the point makes a very narrow loop, as if it is rotating around a half dollar. As you get better, the tip travels less and less until it stays there in the air while the hilt makes wide circles. Of course the point of Professor's sword did not move. I was pretty good at it when I learned it, but since have become pretty bad at it. However, I have made progress in sticking lightly to my partner's sword.

He also said that the idea of the sword form was to get the ch'i to the tip of the sword. Another thing he said about the sword form was that it was to develop the hips. Pretend the sword is very heavy by pushing it and following it. Thereby we will become softer and more sensitive.

Chun-yun, not the Doctrine of the Mean

This lesson is not about T'ai Chi, but something he was equally concerned with: Our ability to be good and ethical human beings.

Professor thought it was important that we students improve as human beings as he had been doing all his life. To do this, he gave us the principle of Chun-yun, which he said was an important teaching of Confucius, often wrongly given as the doctrine of the mean. If it was about the mean, he said, it would not have been an important principle. It would not be something that you could spend your life working on and improving. Just being average or the mean was not what Confucius had in mind.

He wanted us to know the principle as he understood it: This was an idea that you could be working on all your life. You should always be considering how your actions stack up against this principle, always improving at leading your life according to this precept.

Professor Cheng's understanding of Chun-yun:

Do not too much,
and not too little,
Do it not too early,
and not too late.
Just do the exact right amount of a thing at the exact right time.

That was how Professor understood Chun-yun, which Chinese scholars had for years, starting in the time of Confucius, considered as the doctrine of the mean. It is easy to see how adding up too little and too much, too early and too late, one might just as easily get the mean as the exact appropriate.

Professor said that it was the exact appropriate that Confucius was aiming at. The mean is merely the average and does not require much thought. The exact appropriate is a principle that even a sage can always work on, always improve. We need to keep this principle in mind as we go through all the days and years of our lives.

IN THE PRESENCE OF CHENG MAN-CH'ING

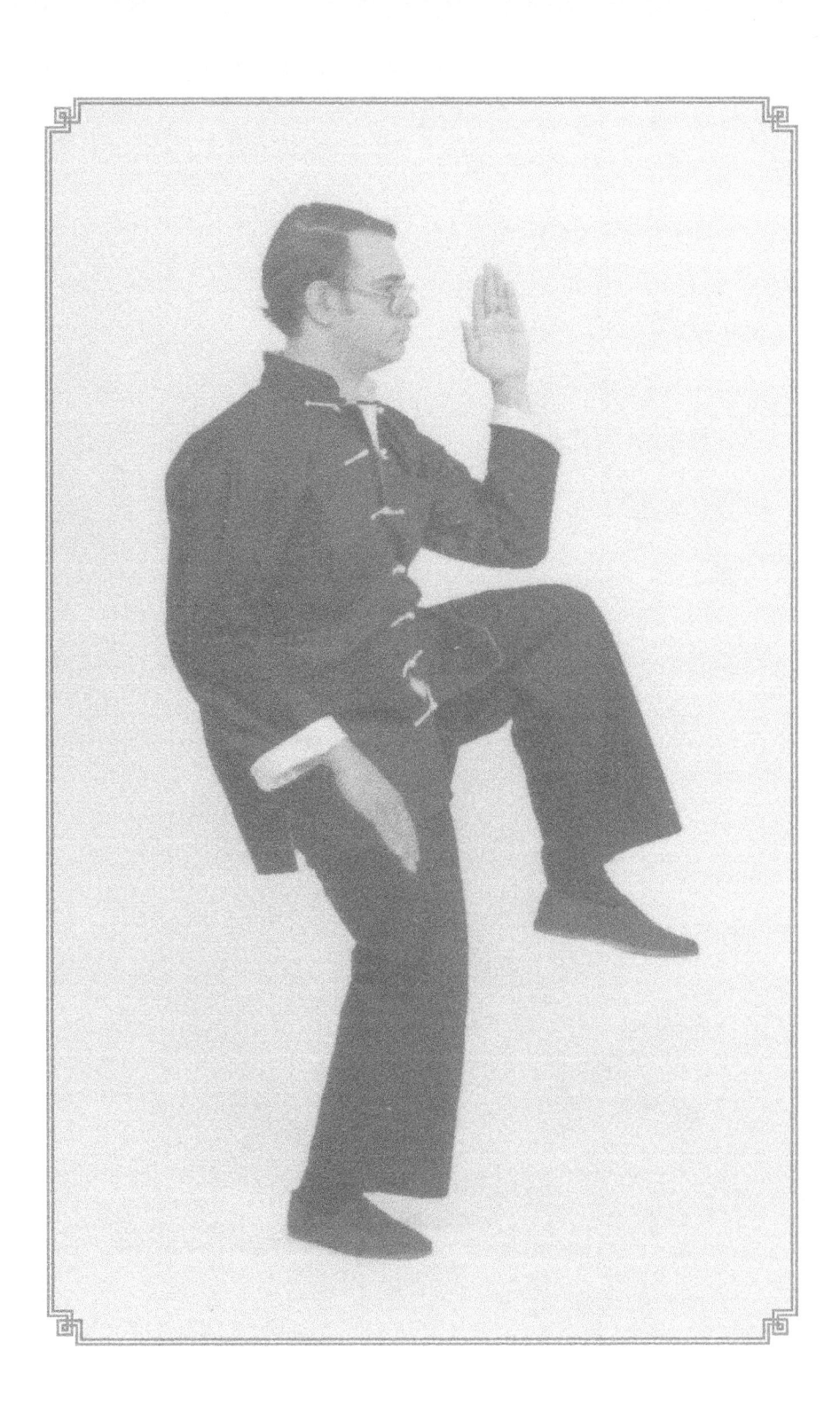

Chapter 12

What I Figured Out for Myself (and with a little help from a friend)

Zhang Lu–Ping (what i did not figure out for myself)

I studied with Master Zhang Lu–Ping from 1988 until his passing in 1998. I am friends with his son, Huan Zhang (American method, family name last) to this day. Lu–Ping taught me some Yang family long form, and mostly improved my push hands. We also shared a lot of fun times. In some of those times we wrote articles together for T'ai Chi Magazine.

He would come to visit on Saturday and stay overnight at my apartment in Brooklyn. Then, on Sunday he would teach a seminar, either at my school, or at a school in Manhattan, or at Princeton. He taught me a lesson on Saturdays. On Sundays he often taught me a little something just before class, to be used that day in the class. He showed me what the lesson for the day in push hands would be as well as the neutralizations, counter pushes and escapes for the pushes, so I could be a proper assistant and not get caught by any of the students.

When we were in Manhattan, he would sometimes review with me on the doorsteps of the schools we would be working at, to make sure I had it. He may have done this because when I was a student, I could defeat all the techniques of most of his assistants. Only he could reliably toss me, and we did not want that to happen again with anyone else.

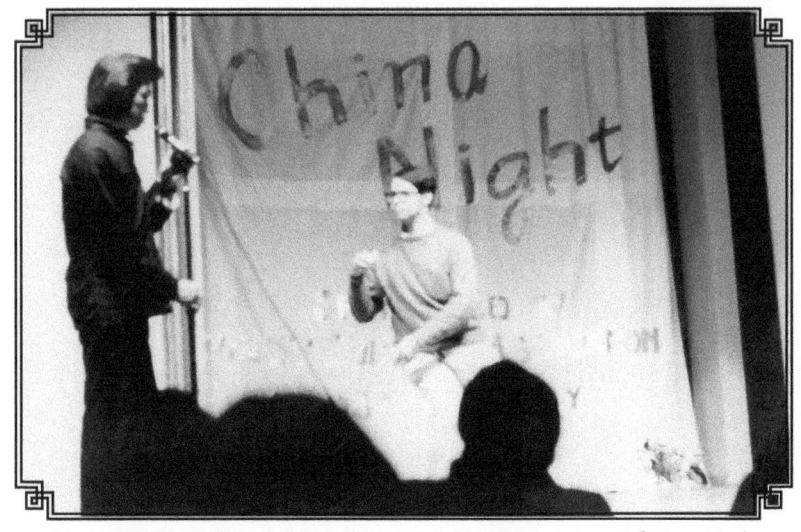

China Night Cultural Festival At The City University Of New York. William C. Phillips demonstrates the t'ai chi form with narration by one of Professor Cheng's sons, Patrick Cheng.

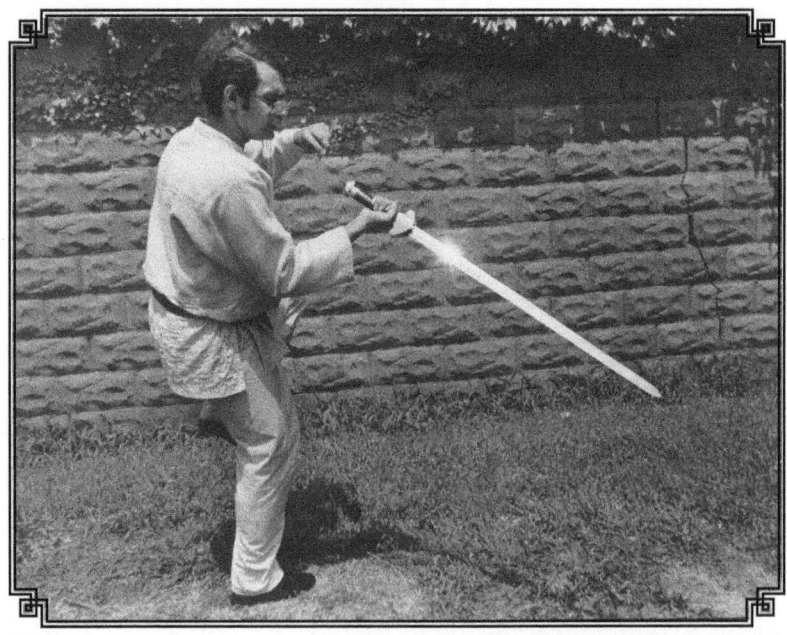

William C. Phillips practicing Professor Cheng's sword form in his back yard in the 1970s. *Photo credit:* Kathy Libraty

IN THE PRESENCE OF CHENG MAN-CH'ING

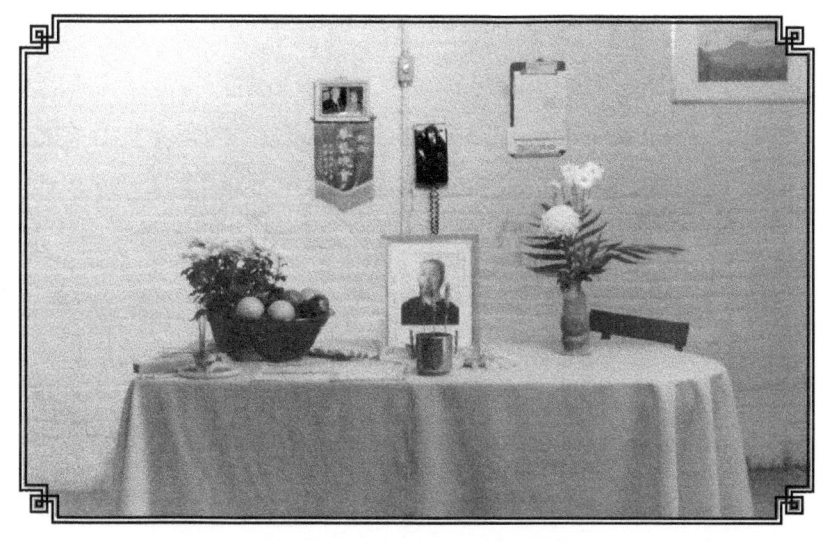

Memorial at the Shr Jung school placed after Professor Cheng passed away in Taiwan, 1975.

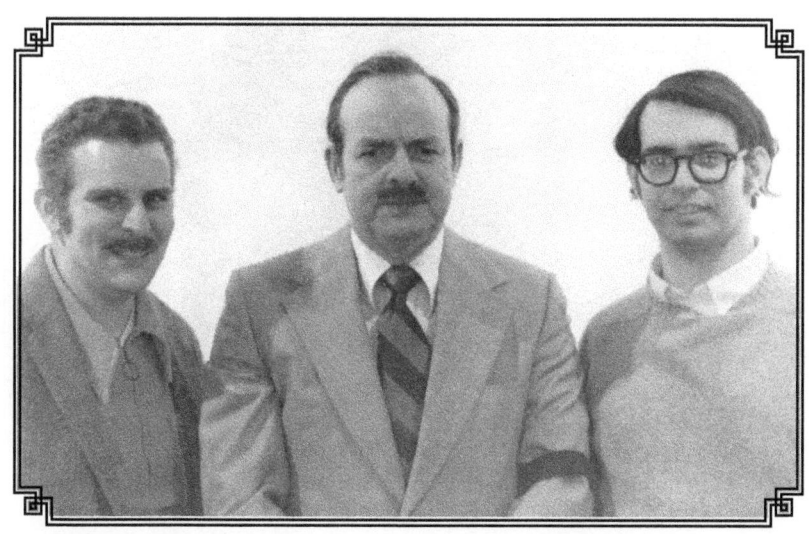

Professor Cheng's first Western student and chronicaller Robert W. Smith with New York students Mort Raphael (left) and William C. Phillips (right).

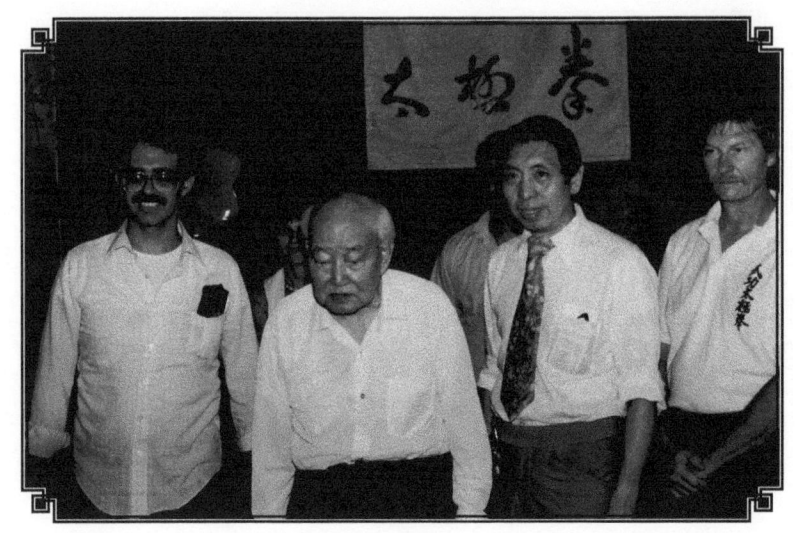

William C. Phillips, T.T. Liang, William C.C. Chen, and Andrew Schirmacher

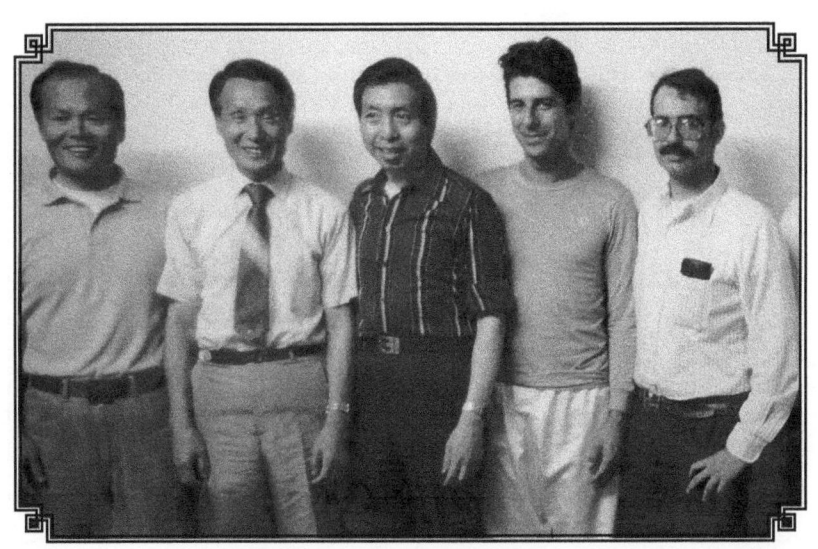

From the left: Benjamin Lo, Jou Tsung Hwa, William C.C. Chen, Robert Morningstar, and William C. Phillips.

IN THE PRESENCE OF CHENG MAN-CH'ING

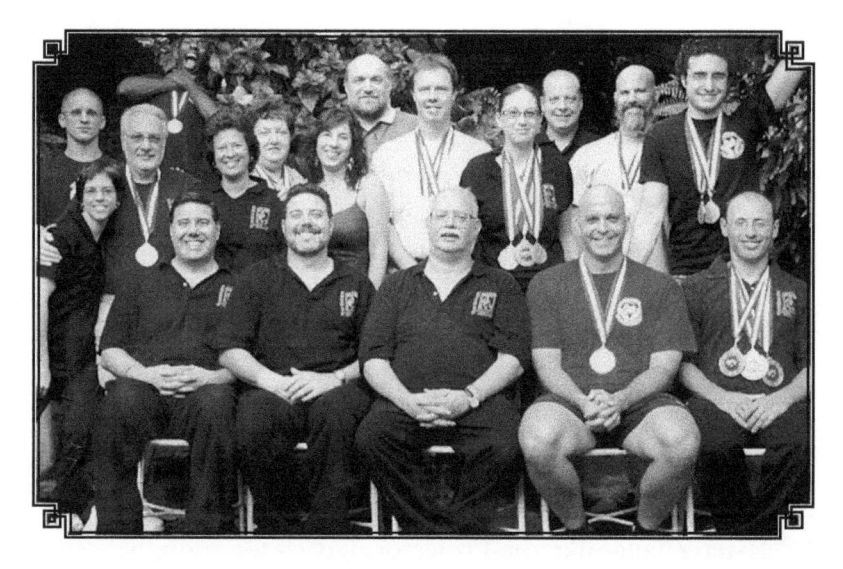

Two schools of Patience T'ai Chi at the Kuo Shu Federation tournament in Maryland. Many won medals. From the left, seated: John Leporati, Jim Lepoprati, and William C Phillips (coaching staff), and Michael Pekor and Avi Schneier. First row standing from left: Elizabeth Crefin, Fred Mirer, Marisa Coluccio, Susan Marmol, Kurt Smailus, Sue Terry, Dave Lillie, Scott Moses. Back row standing: Greg Gotch, Cecil Addison, Frime Kass, Henry Kass, Keith Rowan. Kurt, Dave, Scott, Greg and Cecil were Mike's students.

When Zhang Lu-Ping came to my school from the People's Republic of China, via Pittsburgh, he did not recognize Professor as a great practitioner. As I studied with Master Zhang, he came to understand. He saw the Professor in what he had taught me, as little as I may have been able to understand. He said that he could teach me to become essentially hard because Professor had taught me to be soft. If I had not learned soft, I could not have learned hard. I would have just interpreted hard as stiff. A number of his other students had that problem.

One of the things I learned from him is how to be hard, and contrast hard with soft. This is an invaluable skill in push hands. He also taught me many ways to push and to neutralize and then counter.

Master Zhang, like the Professor, left us too soon.

Zhang Lu-Ping left me a wonderful picture of himself, one that had been on the altar at his funeral. His wife, Wen Wen, said Lu-Ping wanted me to have it.

In his lifetime, he also asked me to hurry up and write a book, as he wanted to write a forward for me, but I did not write in time for him to do so.

I include a tribute to what he taught me as I begin the part where I write of what I learned, through what I lived, and what I was taught by practice and by life. If I have another book in me, it will be memoirs of my second teacher, and very good friend, Zhang Lu-Ping.

Here's what I learned.

Relaxation

When you have gotten your legs as strong as they will get, by direct assault, it is time to relax. As long as you feel stiff, there is hope. When you feel fine you cannot change, but feeling stiff means that you can relax further. This is a process that will continue all the years of your practice.

Whenever you make a breakthrough, you first experience it as a deficit, then as you achieve (fill that deficit) you feel better. When this no longer happens, and you feel great, then you can worry. Work on your perceived stiffness and weakness, and be of good cheer.

I was told that Ben Lo's calf flapped when he played pushed hands at the Shr Jung, the time he came to visit, and someone slapped it. This happened though he was in a deep stance, with all his weight on that same foot. Such was the nature of his relaxation at that time. Needless to say, I have never achieved that level of leg relaxation.

There are no secrets, but all that is taught is not what it seems.

Most people think Professor had deep secrets, but I found that he did not keep things from us. He wanted us to have them. It is just that his teachings were simple ideas and practices. These simple things needed to be practiced over time for skill to develop. People who saw his great skill chose to think there were more profound and hidden things he was not saying. Things that were easy to understand and could be done with practice were just too simple, in their minds, to be the real reason for his skill. So, they hoped, if only one day he would share his secrets...

I think that many of those people were too stiff and strong to get a lot of what he was trying to explain. Of course, those who could not seem to get it with their first effort, rather than redouble their efforts, chose to think there must be a secret he was not sharing.

Professor said there are no secrets, but he did not say everything was obvious, and it is not. Some of what he taught is hard to accept. Some is not hard to accept or understand, but it is just hard to patiently practice.

Too simple is not secret, nor is it secret if the benefit is not quickly apparent, or not logical to the student. These are not secrets. As an example, Professor said to relax. That was discounted by the logical minds, yet it is of paramount importance to health, to ch'i kung, and to martial art. Some people would rather assume that Professor kept some good stuff secret, than accept what he said: practice and relax. Those that did accept it, developed skill according to their ability.

T'ai Chi, without the sensitivity and awareness that T'ai Chi confers, is just another martial art. So giving away the movements is no great gift without the extras that only practitioners can experience and know.

The operant factor is practice. It's like the joke: One man comes up to another on the platform of the A train in New York City to ask for directions. One asks, "How do I get to Carnegie Hall?" His answer, "Practice, buddy, just practice."

In the same vein, knowing and doing are two different things.

It is like the difference between learning about eating green vegetables for your health and actually eating them daily. Knowing the word T'ai Chi will confer no special benefits, only practice will.

To shamelessly continue, and get practical: A bad round is better than no round. The discipline of practice makes it easier to do all the time. If you were to say, "I am too sick to practice" or "too tired" or "too rushed", it will take less effort to skip your practice next time. You are doing something important for yourself, beyond the T'ai Chi, by practicing the T'ai Chi through adversity.

The discipline of practice makes it easier to do the form all the time. Even if you experience no apparent improvement in your form, and most of us see no improvement from day to day, practice will help you with your self-discipline, which is important to you, whether you can see it or not.

Eventually, the form becomes like candy. It is a desert that caps off your day, and a pre-breakfast treat that starts off your day on just the right note. Then you have to find something else to use as a tool for self-discipline. T'ai Chi will have become a pleasure that you look forward to every morning and night.

Leg tense and stressed should not mean shoulder tension

When your legs are in a state of fatigued leg pain, the pain will rise into the shoulders and make them tense. This is expected, and you need to work at relaxing those shoulders. To be clear, the shoulders need to be relaxed, even while the legs are tense and fatigued, as you work to strengthen the legs.

This will help you with your bodily control as well as your self-discipline. It will further help when you play push hands, to over come and win. If you are ever in a fight and cannot call upon a referee for a needed break, its practical application can be the margin between winning and losing, and thereby suffering more serious pain or injury.

70 – 30

Shifting the weight to seventy percent forward with thirty percent on the back foot is an important principle of T'ai Chi.

To get the weight over the bubbling well of the front foot, do this:

- Put the weight on the rear heel.
- Then shift the weight to the bubbling well and the balls of the rear foot.
- This will push a lot of the weight into the front heel. You will be double weighted.
- Then push the front bubbling well down to become single weighted again.

Your weight should now be approximately seventy-thirty in the front foot.

To test this, see if you can lift the back foot without bobbling your head up and down. Your head may need to travel a bit forwards, but not bobble up and down. The foot will not stay off the floor for long, as you have thirty per cent of your weight over it. But it should come up, briefly, without you needing to move your head upward.

Balance is mostly mental, most of the time

Balance is a good part mental:

If I were to place a 12-inch wide board on the ground, you would probably easily be able to walk across it without any balance problem.

Lift that board to the top of a pair of skyscrapers, and it suddenly is not so easy.

Your balance is, mostly, all in your mind.

Practice slowly

How slowly should you practice?

When you feel that you are going on forever, you are at the gate. When you feel you can go on forever, you have arrived.

Legs and sweat

If you strengthen legs and do not sweat:

You are taking a stance that is too high. If you do not exercise your legs, you may not sweat, as you are not working hard enough.

You may be very fit, in which case a deep stance is not tiring you out yet. Stay there and you will sweat. Have faith.

You may be very relaxed. In which case, you can teach me.

My advice about ch'i (my song of ch'i):

You can move and experience your ch'i.

You say you cannot, but keep it simple.

Energy follows thought.
So if you were really good, you could think it.
Tension blocks energy.
So if you do not have it, relax.
If you think you are relaxed,
relax more.
If you relax enough and let it happen,
relax more, it will.
But you say, I have been relaxing and letting it happen
and it won't.
To you I have two things to say:
Relaxation is a process,
don't stop.
You will become more relaxed, it will help your ch'i to flow.

And the big one:

We all have ch'i in our bodies,
 It is how we feel things like pain, and pleasure.
What else makes your heart beat?
To control the ch'i you have to practice.
It's like saying, man can lift 350 pounds.
Yes he can, you see it at the Olympics every four years.
But if you try, you do not get too far.
The missing ingredient is practice.

So, sow

If you started out with 15 pounds and practiced twice a day, for years, and lifted more when it got easy, eventually you would get to lifting 350 pounds.

And everyone can lift 15 pounds.

Same with ch'i. If you do your practice twice a day for enough years, you will get better at moving ch'i.

If at the same time you are relaxing as much as you can every day and getting better at it, you are preparing the channels to not block the ch'i.

Then when you have done enough work, voila, ch'i.

T'ai chi for ch'i, what I feel

What T'ai Chi gives me is the feeling of improved blood and ch'i circulation. Warmth (circulation) and tingling (ch'i) in the fingers and hands. It is not the tingling like when your hands go to sleep. This tingling is energy, and makes the hands more alert and energetic. Sometimes, but not always, they become so hot it is like hot ice and you cannot tell if it is very hot or very cold. This does not often happen, but when it does it is memorable.

Form for benefits

T'ai Chi is relaxing. When our style is done as it should be done, it is one of the best ch'i kung exercises as well as a good meditation. Many postures have health benefits.

What is necessary is that you do it slowly and smoothly and keep your mind empty of all thoughts while you practice, and that you breathe to the tan t'ien, slowly and smoothly.

Grin and Bear it

Constant Bear is an arm swinging exercise. It is not about how hard you can hit your body, but that your arms are relaxed enough to hit your body. It is also the issue of pushing the ground with the foot and driving the hips around while keeping the arms relaxed. How hard you hit yourself is a function of these things.

Books, including this one, can point the way but cannot replace a teacher.

You need a good teacher, because there are things in the form that you cannot learn from a book. For example: In the brush knee posture the root changes from the back to the front foot, much like a karate reverse punch. To just picture the root in the front foot is like taking a still picture of a racing car going over the finish line. The picture is accurate, but very misleading as to what is actually going on.

Music and T'ai Chi

Slow, long flute tones are fun, especially when doing T'ai Chi. But it is not good for your practice, especially when you are a beginner. T'ai Chi without music can help you focus where you need to focus—in your body:

Feel your body, and there are many things to feel.

Be aware of the environs in which you find yourself, both the physical environment, as well as anyone else in the room.

The latter is the beginning of T'ai Chi as a martial art. This is the way to go. Music lets you go with the flow, and then when you find that your consciousness is carried on the music, you become less aware of the passage of time and of your environs.

Professor said, "Do not let the T'ai Chi do you, you do the T'ai Chi."

You can get to the point where the music does the form with

your body and you do not do the form. You will know you have made this mistake if you get to the end of the form, and have no memory of how you got there.

However, when you have learned the lessons of being aware of yourself and are working on being aware of your environs, music can be part of those environs. At this point you can profit by the music. How, you ask? By not paying it any mind. Be aware of it, and then ignore it at the same time. Do not let it make any patterns for you. You have to be the master of your patterns.

Masters, are we masters?

Sometimes in our training we are going towards a mini peak, and we think we are heading for the top of the mountain. When we get there, and when we look back, we may think we have mastered it. But if we turn around and look the way we are going, we can see the mountain stretches on beyond us, to new heights. If there is a fog, we might think we have mastered it anyway. But sooner or later the fog clears and we can see where we have to go. So more correction, more practice, more work. Always more work.

If we ever do get to the point where we think we may have everything right, maybe we will be true masters. But maybe we will become stagnant for lack of being able to see where our mountain continues to rise.

The three levels commentary

So, you may ask, why do some people think they are masters and show so little skill? I think this is attributable to the three levels.

If you think you are doing it perfectly, you will just keep on doing what you were doing, and not improve. Those of little skill, who think they are masters, are, in my opinion, stuck at the second level.

At the first level, the student needs to be under the tutelage of his master. He needs correction because his form will deteriorate without correction. His form is always deteriorating when he is without instruction to reinforce what is correct. This is because the student does not have the patterns of the movement in his head or in his body. These people do not ever consider themselves masters.

At the second level, the student has finally achieved a certain amount of knowledge and muscle memory, and, therefore, will be able to do it as he was taught. He has the memory, but does not understand the techniques. While he will not get worse, he will not improve. And importantly, he does not understand where the principles of his art can take him. Sometimes these people will decide they are masters. This is because they have the moves, but cannot see where they can be taken, the next level.

At the third level, the student has done the movements and, through good teachers or good look (not luck), he understands them. He can measure what he does against his ideal. He is working on improving at incarnating the principles. The principles are firmly in his consciousness, so he can see how to improve. Then he can improve with practice. This is what Master Jou Tsung Hwa meant when he said the form can teach you.

Form into push hands

Pay attention. It is an important element of the form. It is one of the bridges to self-defense. First, be aware of your body, really aware, of exactly where your weight is, your arms and legs and spine and knees and elbows. When you really know where your body is, then be aware of your environment during the form.

During push hands, be aware of yourself and also your opponent or partner. Finally, in push hands be aware of yourself, your partner and the space you are in, your external environment. Then you are transitioning to the martial.

Push Hands

If done properly, push hands reinforces your understanding of the form. It also teaches real softness. If you think you are soft and you bend or knock down a small tree when you encounter one slowly as you do your form, or are stopped by the tree, you are not soft. So when you think you are soft and are found rigid by a partner, your partner has done you a service by finding you tense or rigid. Thank him/her.

Yield and Neutralize

These terms do not mean the same thing. Yield means to get out of the line of force with no resistance. Whether you withdraw until the force is spent or you sit to a side is not important to the term. However, while you can yield without neutralizing, you cannot neutralize without yielding. Yielding does not imply getting a superior position, neutralizing does.

When you neutralize, you yield with a purpose. The purpose is to get a superior position, whether to dissipate the attack, to let the person fall over himself, or to prepare to push, or issue force.

Push Hands and Listening

Push hands teaches you about listening skills, which is an important part of T'ai Chi. It also teaches you the value of being in the here and now. This will help you to use form as an awareness exercise as well as a meditation and not get lost in it.

Push

Issuing force is used in T'ai Chi, often called a fa chin (fajin) or jing, a springy force that comes from pressing the floor with your foot. When you do, it comes back up the legs through the hips to the hands to forcefully push someone away. It is typically done after a neutralization, when the person is off balance and/or leaning into you, therefore presenting a good target. But if your hands are not relaxed, you will be losing some of the force and not transmitting it all to your opponent. This force is the stuff of the no-inch and one-inch punches and can be done through hands that are not particularly relaxed. The more you relax, the more efficiently you will be able to transmit force, and the more powerful this technique will become.

I rarely push with "jing". I try to feel, to sense my partners and then gently off-balance them. I use listening skills most of the time. Occasionally I make a little tension and then push into that. I try to not use "jing". But then I do not wish to hurt my students. Like anything else, not practicing, it gets weaker. But like riding a bike, once you have it, it does not go completely away.

Swords

The sword form is learned moving slowly through the postures, like the form. When you know the postures, you may want to learn the sword form again, in a different way.

You push the sword and follow it, moving at the appropriate speed of the movement of your sword. This requires you to develop a sensitivity to your sword. It is often here where people start to see the light in T'ai Chi.

I recommend heavy swords in correction for those who are using their hands and wrists to control the sword. If that is the case, they need a sword so heavy that they cannot control it, and then they have to do the form by pushing the sword and following it, using the waist, which is how the sword form should be done.

After that, and as long as you practice, your sword should feel light in your hand.

WILLIAM C. PHILLIPS

The Best Advice I Have for You, Unasked For

Professor made me feel like I was a part of his family. And so I did my best to make my own T'ai Chi and martial arts students my family.

Here are some questions and answers (maybe covering the same ground, maybe with a new insight).

What Does It Mean to Be Relaxed?

It is a process. If you relax on day one, and do the same relax a year later, that is not relaxed anymore, unless you have made no progress.

You relax as much as possible every day and it gets better as you continue to relax.

Keep in mind, being dead weight (collapsed) is not being relaxed. Relaxed is being light and alert, sensitive to movement and light enough to follow, like a summer suit you are wearing.

What Is Meant by the Saying: "Invest in Loss"?

If you cannot overcome with T'ai Chi principle, then get pushed, get beaten. But do it wisely. Learn from the experience, so that in the next time or two you do not make the same mistake. Sooner or later, with the right mind, you will eventually run out of mistakes and figure out how to use T'ai Chi principles to overcome and then you will no longer lose.

How does one sink the ch'i to the tan t'ien?

Breathe it there, and feel it. You do not have lungs there, so it is ch'i that you are feeling. If it is not going there, be patient and stay relaxed. Eventually it will, if you persist in a relaxed way. Why do it? You do it because it is storing energy, and it feels good. Also it will bring ch'i to the hands and feet, which also feels good. It may help to keep your extremities warm in cold weather.

Rooting, foothold. How do you sink your center of gravity into the floor?

I can teach you, but then again, I have to show you. I cannot do this in writing. The transmission is physical. I would have to set you up and then, if you are relaxed enough, you will feel it and maybe do it. It is about forty percent relaxation, fifty-five percent right posture, and maybe five percent ch'i. This is just an approximation. You cannot do it without relaxation, even if you have the right posture. You cannot do it without right posture, even if you have the relaxation.

Neutralizing an attack, any tips?

Yes, practice the form, feel the air. Then practice push hands with a partner. It will come slow but it will come. If you can feel the air, how much more substantial will any partner be.

How do I control my ch'i?

Breathe to the tan t'ien, and relax while doing so. Even better, practice T'ai Chi while breathing to the tan t'ien, including the inhales and exhales of the form. First you have to feel it. Then try to get it to go where it was going, but faster, or stronger. Finally, you may try to move it where it was not going, and thereby control it.

Use four ounces to deflect a thousand pounds?

Yes. Many students worship and are very reverential about this statement. It is not mystical. When you are sensitive and can catch someone by their balance, it does not take much more than four ounces to push him/her along the line of their off-balance. Pushing in other directions takes a lot of strength. But following the line of off-balance is almost effortless. Of course this does not work on dead weight, like statues for example.

If you are relaxed enough, you can feel your partner searching for your off-balance points, and he will not find them, and you will smile. Four ounces will not work with you.

What do I pay attention to?

I pay attention to everything. As I mentioned earlier, it is an important element of the form. It is one of the bridges to self–defense. First, be aware of your body, really aware, of exactly where your weight is, your arms, elbows and wrists, and legs, hips and ankles, and the straightness of your spine. See that knees and elbows work together. Feel your breath, your ch'i, how your head is suspended from above. Be aware of how you are moving, softly, and with your head on one level. When you really know where you are, then be aware of your environment during the form. Be aware of your partner, and his internal space (Where is he off balance, for example). Finally in push hands be aware of your partner and his spacing from you and the space you both are in, your external environment.

IN THE PRESENCE OF CHENG MAN-CH'ING

My wisdom, just a bit of it since I am the author

He who knows not,
and knows not that he knows not,
is a fool,
Shun him.

He who knows not,
and knows that he knows not,
is a student,
Teach him.

He who knows,
and knows not that he knows,
is asleep,
Awaken him.

He who knows,
and knows that he knows,
is wise.
Follow him.

And some wisdom from other teachers, I think is important

Yard by yard, Life is hard
Inch by inch, Life's a cinch
—Al Casuto

What you fight, will fight you back.
And bring you misery, suffering and lack.
But when you learn to go with the flow,
Both good, and bad, will help you grow.

— Iz Freidman

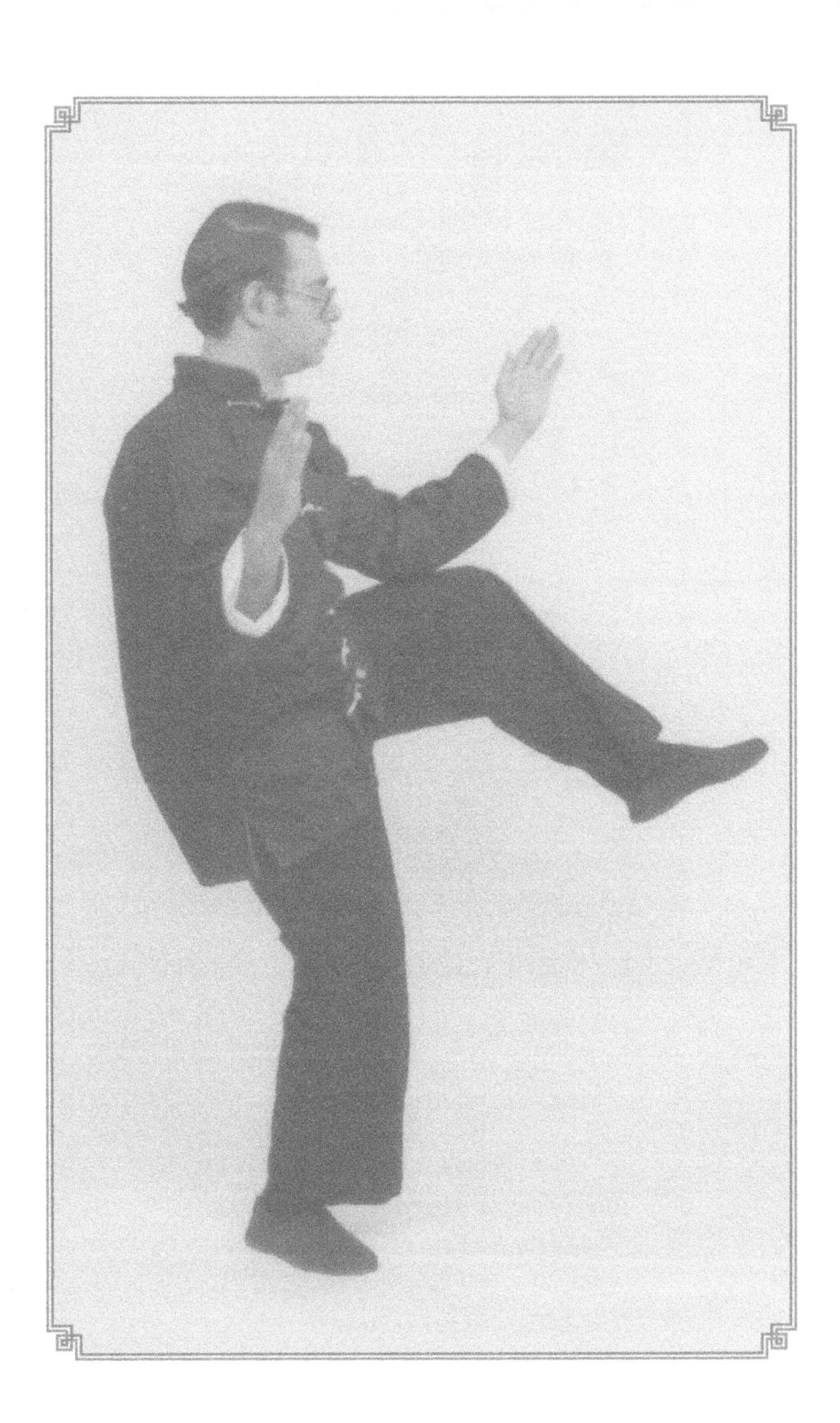

Chapter 13

Self–Defense

I taught the martial arts I had learned, or figured out, from 1970 to 1993. I had some incidents before that, as a student, and many more during that period. I used what I learned and taught in real situations, too many to recount here, but I will list a few here, to give the flavor of the times I lived in.

While I had a back injury in 1980, I recovered from it and continued to train. After my arm injury in 1993, the hospital must have dropped me on my back while I was unconscious, as it was unstable ever after until very recently. I was unable to continue training, at first, beyond the T'ai Chi form. After some time I was able to add some push hands. Now I walk and lift light weights, I try not to push myself too hard, something that is always a danger. I want to get back to martial training if my age has not caught up with me and made it impossible. I will keep doing what I can do, until I cannot do it any longer.

I want to say that I did not write this chapter out of ego. My students were curious, and so I thought the readers would be as well. I should say here that I never did learn the T'ai Chi "applications" but applied the principles of T'ai Chi to the martial arts I had already learned. That has stood me in good stead until my final injury stopped me from doing what I had been doing. I want to emphasize that I have no special skill, except that imparted by T'ai Chi and my teachers. So if I can do these things, all my readers can as well.

Let me also say that fighting was not the purpose of any of my T'ai Chi training. Self-perfection was my goal. But I have to admit that the martial came in handy numerous times in my life and in my work.

I will start with a sparring incident, not a fight at all.

Chin, or jing lesson

I figured out "fa chin" or "jing," for pushing or the no-inch punch. It is the same principle. It really is kind of simple if you are relaxed and can make your body into one unit (hard) and push the ground with a foot, letting the force rise. I used to practice it on heavy bags, putting my hand against it and making it fly.

Once, when I was sparring, I hit someone with a couple of open snap strikes in the face, and he kept coming. That usually did not happen. I straightened my right hand into a fist and just as he got close, I no-inch punched him in the rib cage. I was surprised at what happened. My fist did its thing and he did not move, instead his rib cage bent from the pressure of my hand. Then as his rib cage re-expanded, he went flying back. When I explained what it felt like to someone who saw it and wondered at the delay in the explosion of power, they pointed out that if I had hit the floating rib I might have killed my student. I decided not to do that, ever again.

I avoided injuring people with the no-inch kick. I used to put my foot up against the bag, and then make it fly, same principle. At work they had these big, two hundred pound or so (by my estimate) doors. A couple of them were warped, so they could only be opened with leaning and a good push. I would walk at the doors and raise my foot to open them. One day a student thought that it was interesting and wanted to see if I could open it without the momentum of walking, I put my foot against the door and blasted it open so hard it hit the wall and bounced back.

In my street fights I used a slow version of that kick to just gently push attackers back, but once, when my attacker had help on the way, I blasted him with it (as you will see below).

IN THE PRESENCE OF CHENG MAN-CH'ING
CHALLENGES IN T'AI CHI PUSH HANDS

When, in 1993, I told Stanley that I was going to enter the Taste of China tournament, he asked me, "What do you have to prove?" He then answered his own question and said, "You have nothing to prove." I did not listen (a major fault of mine even then). I would have gone into the event except that I was prevented from doing so. My biceps tendon snapped that year in June and the event was the following month. The surgery ended my competitive days in judo, karate, ju jitsu, and push hands.

That June of 1993, before the injury, I was teaching a seminar on my beginners' neutralization exercises, at the Zhang San Feng Festival at Master Jou Tsung Hwa's T'ai Chi Farm. I was working on the main dirt roadway, beyond the Zhang Building before the road wended its way into the forest. Students were sitting on the rise on one side of the road and standing in the drop on the other side.

I called for volunteers at various points of the seminar and asked that they push in a particular way so I could demonstrate each principle I was discussing. A guy stepped out in answer to one of my calls for a helper. I asked him to gently push my left hand, in and around to the left, as I had my right foot back. It was my intention to demonstrate a neutralization from that side of the body, the same side as the front foot. This is important because it is harder to do than the other side of the body, the side of the back foot. I wanted to demonstrate that you can turn the hip in that direction, "the hard side," as well as the side of the foot that is back, "the easy side." It was an exercise I had designed to increase flexibility and neutralization skill in the tradition of Mort Raphael who created so many exercises for me.

As I offered my arm to his two hands, he quickly pushed straight back, in and up, into my chest, instead of in the direction I had asked him to push. I think he intended to trap my arm to my chest and push me straight over my rear heel. But, reflexes engaged, I dropped away from him into a squatting single whip (also known as snake creeps up, or down), letting his hands take my arm where he intended it to go. He intended it to go into my chest, but with me dropping down, it went directly over my head.

He was surprised to find himself leaning over me, as he apparently expected my arm to be connected to my chest at that point. Instead, it was loosely attached to nothing much beyond a very flexible shoulder, and going exactly where he was pushing it.

Then I came back from the squatting single whip, placing my right hand on his ribs as I rose into him by straightening my back leg. I caught him square in his chest, on an upward angle, with my right hand connected to my right foot, rooted solidly to the ground. He went about a foot in the air, three feet back and bounced.

I like to think that I was thought to be pretty good by those who had eyes to see what had happened. I hoped they knew that this was not planned. I had been sneakily attacked.

That gentleman went on to win the Taste of China tournament that year. I went on to be hospitalized with a torn right biceps tendon. My competitive push hands career, over.

But back to the story: I continued, without missing a beat for those watching. I made a comment about being given the opportunity to show some different techniques than I had intended to teach. I then asked him to push gently around the hard side, and he did.

God gave me these opportunities, God and good reflexes.

Another challenge happened when I was not teaching but just hanging around at the T'ai Chi Farm. A woman sifu thought she could beat me, but had the decency to take me out behind the Zhang building to try me, so that I might not be beaten and humiliated in front of every one. I won that one as well, I could neutralize her pushes, and she could not push me. We are lifelong friends to this day.

Another time a famous teacher needed someone to push to demonstrate a point he was making. He called me over asked me if I would be part of a teaching demonstration with him, and when I said OK, he told me to neutralize if I could. He pushed, I neutralized, he tried again, and again, I neutralized again and again. At length, he realized I was not so easy to push. At that point, he asked me to cooperate so he could demonstrate his technique. We also are friends to this day.

This actually happened twice, with two different masters, both now friends. But as the story is roughly the same, consider it told.

At the Kuo Shu tournament, long after my injury, as I was starting on the long road back, the woman who became a lifelong friend after challenging me at the T'ai Chi Farm brought two Chinese masters to try me in successive years.

One gentleman told me he wanted to try me as I was standing by the outdoor pool. He put a foot forward, and tried to push. I neutralized and returned a push. He was off-balanced, but held on to my shirt for balance, and so we both went flying back into a poolside vinyl chair. With me on top, since he held on to me, he made a comfortable mat to land on.

The other guy met me in a hallway. When he could not push me, he tried a technique which I know as kuba nage, its Japanese name.

He put an arm around my neck and turned and tried to throw me over his leg. If I had not had judo training it probably would have worked. I ducked out of the throw and pushed him away from me. It seemed to me he wanted to fight, and kuba nage, to me, is not push hands. So I got into a stance and ready. Fortunately, that was the end of the incident.

My students, Avi Schneier and Mike Pekor wanted to play with him and show him what they were about, in defense of me. They beat him roundly, and came to tell me about it. While I bent my neck and let his hand fly by me, over my head, Mike stuck his arm across the guy's neck when he tried it with him, and peeled him off. He has photos of that.

The last story of a challenge is foolish really. A student of mine, a woman at that, got it into her head that I was a master (which I do not claim) and could, if attacked, defeat her without really pushing her or hurting her. So one day, without warning, she attacked. My reflexes engaged and she got pushed away, several feet and landed on her butt. She blamed me and said a master could take a challenge and not defeat his students. I never said I was a master. And I do not know where she got the idea that she could surprise attack me and I could defend myself and not hurt her.

One further story: I was told of an incident I did not even remember. The husband of a student put his hand on my shoulder to get my attention. It was not as a challenge. He was about 6'3" and about 300 lb. My reflexes were engaged, and somehow, he went flying across the floor, a victim of those reflexes.

Tournaments

It was not for me to play in tournaments, I had to leave that to my students. Two stories come to mind:

Let me tell you of the time I used perfect principle to win a championship, and then they withdrew the championship trophy. Once, in the '70s, at a tournament in New Jersey, in the dan ranked ju jitsu division, I was preparing to compete. I stretched and warmed up, not a characteristic thing for me to do, but I was bored. All my potential competitors saw what I was doing, and every one of them withdrew, so the promoters refunded my money and did not award the trophy.

Another incident of interest happened at a tournament in Brooklyn in the '80s. A student of mine was having some words and difficulties with a group of teens from another school. He was in front of them, coaching our students. They wanted him to "Sit down in front" so they could see. In truth, he could not sit and still do a good job for Patience T'ai Chi. They said they would beat his ass (a common Brooklyn refrain of hostility) for not getting out of their line of sight. At length, he went to the bathroom and I got a funny feeling that I should follow him. Just then the teenagers left their seats. I left also and followed them. As my student started using the urinal, the group took positions directly behind him. I walked over to a position directly behind them and crossed my arms. I felt feelings of protectiveness towards my student and extreme hostility towards them. They looked at him, looked nervously behind themselves at me, looked at each other and left. I won without fighting.

Fights

Once, when I was Nikkyu (2nd Brown), I had a fight with a friend of a house plan brother. It lasted about two seconds. He said, "So you think you know karate," took a stance and attacked. I kicked him in the ankle, with a low side kick, breaking the ankle. End of fight. No fancy hollering, or punching or foot work, just a swift low kick to the ankle. End of story.

In the 1970s, on the street, I was attacked by a rather hot-tempered man over a parking space I did not even want. He honked at me when I was double-parked and so I pulled into the spot, thinking he was not a confident driver and just wanted to go around me. I thought that I was blocking him. But he wanted the spot, little did I know.

Anyway, he parked around the corner, and walked back past me. As he came by, across the street, he started cursing at me. I turned to look at him, out of the driver's side window, and said "Same to you," dismissively, and turned to face the windshield again. My mistake. He attacked. As he came for the car, swinging, I got out of the car. He threw an over-handed, over-his-head punch at me. I blocked him with a rising block. He repeated this several times more, and several times more I defended with a rising block. Finally, after blocking this persistent gentleman, I gently kicked, more of a push than a kick, to push him away. I used a slow front thrust kick, as he did not seem to be getting tired of attacking. After a few of these interactions, I saw a group of his friends coming and I thought I would have to fight them all. So when the gentleman came back even stronger, I forcefully kicked him cleanly over the hood of my 1970 Barracuda. He was about three or four feet in front of the car. He flew back. His buttocks were raised over the hood by the lift of the kick, and his thighs raised parallel to the hood and he slid back. Next, his knees came up over the hood with the power of the kick, and he slid entirely across the hood and fell on the far side of the car. He got up, but he was wobbly, and he was no longer aggressive. I turned to face his friends, and they, instead of joining the fight, gathered around my assailant, and took him away. They called me crazy, which was fine with me, as long as there was no continuation of the fight.

Another time, in the evening, I was cut off on the highway. I cut the person off right back and did not think any more of it. He followed me off the highway and ran me off the road and tried to "kick my ass," as he said. I rising blocked and softly kicked him until he gave up and drove off. This time, with no friends coming, I was able to take my time and let him wear out and quit. I did not have to get to any really rough stuff. I should point out two things one good and one not so good: First, the not so good: I knocked my glasses off with my own rising block; Second, the good, I did not realize this, and continued with no apparent loss of vision. So intent was I on what I was doing, that I did not notice that I did not have my glasses on until after, when I got back into my car to drive away. Then I was unable to see to drive.

Almost a fight, almost an opponent.

One time I was walking across Avenue X in the West streets in Brooklyn, coming from the pork store. I walked across the street towards the elementary school, on a frigid windy day. As the street was icy, I was walking hunched over and knees bent so I could better keep my balance. When I got to the other side of the street, I straightened up. I immediately felt someone, or something (as it turned out) hitting my head. My reflexes engaged, and I did a forward aikido roll to evade my attacker. When I got up, facing, in a defensive stance, I saw that I had straightened up, after crossing the street, right into a school bus mirror. That was what had "hit me" in the head. After that, I also noticed that I'd torn my jeans and hit my knee pretty hard, and it began to hurt. Though, when I thought I might have been under attack, so focused was I, I felt nothing.

A challenge but not a fight.

In 2018, at the New Life Expo, as I was volunteering for Gail Thackray, a guy came up to me and said I looked familiar. He also said I lost weight, which told me he did not really know me as I had not, up to then. I told him I did T'ai Chi and he put a foot forward, and so I put one back, and he pushed, straight and hard. I neutralized two of those pushes, so he came back with some wing chun moves, and still I neutralized. So he came back with punches. I blocked three and slapped him on his head. At this point security from the hotel, as well as security for the event, had converged on us, perhaps thinking that a real fight was taking place. I have to admit, that is what it looked like. Event security, who had seen me around and knew me, said, "Shhhh, calm down." I grabbed the guy to me and said "Enough." But he was not listening, so I raised my right foot in a very constricted round-house chambered position, my knee to his chest, to keep him from trying to hit me. He stopped.

We then talked for a while. He said the he had gotten out of line like that with Master Goldberg, and he had gotten hit in the head for his troubles. He said that he knew I was the real deal.

I had to go but before I left, event security told me we were acting like a couple of kids. End of story.

Work issues

I was Student Cafeteria Coordinator for five periods a day, and later School Security Coordinator, also for five periods a day. On the one hand, officially we were told not to mix it up with the students, to call security guards. Unofficially, I was told to maintain order, and do whatever was necessary to do so. I did that job from the early 1970s until October 3, 1980. During that time I would fight once or twice a week, in the student cafeteria.

I would occasionally fight in the hallways and in the classrooms. Most of those fights were not about maintaining order, but about breaking up fights. You see, often one of the two kids engaged in a fight did not want to fight. I felt I had to help those kids. Often, when I inserted myself in between the students, the aggressor would start to try to hit me. And I would block and do whatever was appropriate to stop him. After a while I developed a strategy for those kids. I stepped into the middle and grabbed the kid who did not want to fight by the shoulders, and pushed him back. I then threw a high side kick in front of the head of the other kid. I did this much more quickly than it takes to tell. When the other kid saw my foot, and that his target was out of range, he usually calmed down and the fight was over. I did not actually kick any kids, though occasionally aggressive students walked right into my foot.

Lest I give the wrong impression, my actual fights at work were messy things, martial arts or not. At least to me they were. My street fights were with people who, while furious, were not particularly fast or skilled. At work, they were fast, somewhat skilled, and worst of all for me, experienced. So after each incident, I would analyze what had happened and, back at the dojo, train to fight that fight better if that situation ever came up again. As is the nature of fights, it very rarely happened, so I kept training new situations as they arose. I also drilled basics. I hope I kept my martial arts students entertained.

Once I was shot at. I was not a hero. I turned, ran, and did a forward roll over a cafeteria table, caught it with a foot and pulled it down behind me. Fortunately, at that time, we had the old tables that were not connected to the chairs. I then crawled along the table, out of sight of the kid, so that if he put another shot where I was, I would no longer be there. He did not shoot again. Not being a trained marksman, his only shot was high and, later, I saw the hole in the ceiling tile above and beyond where I had been. That was where the bullet went. I do not think it was his intention to shoot me, but merely to stop me from breaking up the fight I came over to break up, as his friend was winning. After the shot, they both ran out of the cafeteria. Such is the nature of a gun barrel pointing at you that I do not know if I ever saw either of them again.

Other times I occasionally disarmed kids, taking knives away from them. I was not the target of their anger, so it was easy, especially if I knew the kid. We had a school police officer and I left the taking of guns to him. That activity was beyond my pay grade.

These are a few of the incidents that happened in the school cafeteria:

Often I had a student who wanted to run over me to get out of the student cafeteria without a pass. One time, I had a curious fight over this issue. It was my job to stop him. As we were moving, and he was jabbing at the air in front of me, as we faced off, we turned gradually around so that he had his back to the door. He could have just turned and run out, but he continued fighting.

In those days kids would throw butter patties from their lunch up so they would stick to the ceiling. As I continued to move with him, waiting for my opportunity to hit him and end the fight, one patty fell and it landed right in front of me. As I stepped forward, I slipped on it. As I fell, so as not to lose the fight and face among the rest of the students in the cafeteria, I lunged forward. I grabbed him and fell on top of him at the top of the stairs leading down to the exit. I had cracked my head on the ceiling at the top of the stairs as I fell onto him. I ended the fight by holding his arms and bleeding into his eyes until he quit moving. I then went to the medical office. The student regained his self-control, and actually came by to see if I wanted to have him suspended. I did not, since his attitude had changed and he was no longer acting the tough guy. Otherwise, I would have referred him to the dean for disciplinary action.

That was an example of my sense of justice. According to the school rules, I should have had him suspended and arrested. But I saw no reason to, as he seemed chastened.

One day I heard chaos on the other side of the student cafeteria. One student was chasing another with a 10-inch or so knife (a kitchen knife). I got in between them and grabbed the hand with the knife, since it was outstretched in front of him. I also grabbed the kid's other hand, and suggested he calm down. He was not listening and tried to gut me (my gut was a lot smaller in those days, and fortunately, not so much of a target). As he lunged, I neutralized (got my body out of the way) and then threw him with an osoto gari. As the kid was really strong, I leaned on the knife hand, which I had pinned to his body. I was in kind of a pre-downward dog yoga posture, so all my weight was pushing the knife against his body. A security guard reached between my legs and twisted the knife out of his hand. Eventually, I got letters of commendation from both the Principal (*see Appendix 1*) and the Superintendent of the district for it. It was nice to be seen as doing my job well. But, back at the time it happened, there was no time to congratulate or even compose myself. The bell rang and I had to arrange with security for the student to be taken to the office and deal with the next incoming lunch period.

Another thing that happened, the memory of which I kind of enjoy: In the late 1970s I had a student in the cafeteria whose last name was Phillips, same as mine. One day he wanted to fight with me over something stupid, as was often the case when a fight was being picked with me. I saw little opportunity to use words to avoid it, so I told him to put his hands wherever he wanted, and I would hit him in the face anyway. And if I did hit him, I hoped he would see the futility of fighting with me. He put his hands up and I smacked him right through his hands. He did not believe it though he felt it. He wanted to see that again, and so I obliged. Then he got control of himself and we avoided the fight. I put him on my service squad, and he served loyally and well. He even offered to come to my classes and tell those kids he would kick their asses if they ever messed with me.

I learned lessons as I fought. One time a kid who had a reputation as a very tough fighter, came against me. He was not a big guy, but bigger guys, guys that did not get out of many people's way, warned me that he was a good fighter. They suggested that I stay out of his way. Anyway, he wanted to get out of the student cafeteria, and I was blocking his way. So he threw a punch, and, paying attention to what I had heard, I threw an inside block as fast as I could. I caught some air, and at that point I realized that he was not so very fast, fierce maybe, but not fast. I put my hand down and blocked again, and the second block caught his hand. And he was impressed with me, and stopped. No one had blocked him before. Peace was maintained. The lesson is one of appropriate speed. We train for speed, but to be too fast is as bad as to be too slow. A miss is a miss. I was very lucky, I got a second chance that day, and I know that second chances in a fight are about as rare as hen's teeth.

In case you think I am making myself the hero of these tales, (which I may very well be doing) there is the life-changing event that happened on October 3, 1980 at around 11:00 AM. I know exactly when my role as school security and cafeteria coordinator came to an end. A gang fight broke out in the student cafeteria. It was one gang of Chinese Americans versus two gangs of African Americans. It was my job to keep order and so I ran into the middle of it and tried to stop it.

In this particular fight a lot of chairs were being thrown. Whichever way I turned, my back found another chair. A call went out from our school police officer for help. Police officers, and, as we were downtown, correction officers, and court officers responded. In all it seemed to me that about 100 uniformed officers came to break up that fight. I did not go down, but I felt a weird pain in my back and it did not feel right. So, when the action was over, I went to the medical office and then home. Fortunately I was able to drive myself home before it got worse, and it got a lot worse.

I thought I was in pain. But compared to what was coming, I was a stranger to pain. I had been in an automobile accident in 1965, and hit a tree at about 30 miles per hour. My head had destroyed the windshield, my knee had been cut on the emergency brake, and my arms had broken the steering wheel off its column. The steering column then hit my chest, or rather, my chest hit it, hard. But I had not known pain.

After the fight on October 3, the pain settled in slowly over the course of about two weeks. At first, I could sit for half an hour, then stand for a half hour and then lie down for a half hour and as long as I kept changing position, it did not hurt too much. It just felt weird, and sometimes I had numbness down my legs as well. I was getting more and more sleepy, as I could not sleep for more than half an hour at a time. The pain was my alarm clock. And I had to stand or walk around for half an hour roughly every hour and a half. But the pain was getting worse and worse. My Dad, who influenced how I thought of painkillers, was of the grin and bear it people, and so I did not want painkillers. But that was to change.

Finally, about four weeks after, I got a lift to my martial arts school to watch and direct class, and take my mind off the pain. And something happened. I was sitting on the desk, and I kind of slid off with no muscle control. On the one hand it felt like my back was made of water, nothing holding me up, on the other hand, at the same time it felt like cement, cold and hard and rigid. I was in agony and really found out the meaning of pain from then forward. My students carefully put me in a car and drove me home. They carried me into my house and laid me down on the couch.

Up to that point, I had not been interested in painkillers. I was prejudiced against them, as I mentioned, because of my Dad. When I had broken my collarbone playing judo, I was given a prescription for painkillers. I took one, and when I woke up, I flushed the rest down the toilet. I was afraid of them.

From the minute I fell off that desk, however, I needed them, and needed them badly. When I was asked, many years later, by

Su Terry, a student, if I was ever discouraged by the setbacks of my injuries, inhibiting what I could do, I answered no, I was only discouraged by the pain when I was in it and when it was at its worst, for days on end.

In spite of the many fights I had broken up and the weapons I had successfully taken from students, I got no sympathy or patience from the school. They wanted me back to work, healthy or not, or else I was a malingerer. On December 15 of that year, they ordered me back and took me off the payroll. Because my dad was an attorney, we fought back with legal process, and I was granted a medical arbitration.

The arbitration was in January and I was starting to feel a bit better, admittedly with the help of the painkillers. The arbitration was a curious affair. The doctor asked me to stretch, and when I could just about touch my ankles with my fingertips, he said I had great flexibility. But before the injury, I could put my wrists to the ground behind my heels. He did not care. Finally, he had me lie down on a medical examination table and dropped the end panel so that my legs, from the knees, fell 90 degrees suddenly. I yelped in surprised agony, the painkillers were not working then. As a result of that surprise torture, I won the medical arbitration, but went home in continuing agony. Though I won the arbitration, and was given back pay, I was and told I had to report back to work on a set date, with no further medical leave and no further medical exams. I do not remember the exact date, sometime the end of February, but it was not enough time, especially since the arbitration itself caused renewed pain. But I returned to school, heavily medicated, and stinking from tiger balm.

It took a while but I did eventually recover from that injury. I have the video of me doing stuff to prove it. But when my biceps tendon had to be reattached, and I was knocked out for surgery, they must have dropped me on my back, or somehow aggravated the injury. I say this because my back became painful and unstable. Once again I was not able to do things I wanted to do, and once again I needed painkillers. I have always tried not to let the pain and instability in my back stop me from doing the things I enjoy. But it is now 39 years later and I am still unable to do some things as a result of that injury. Randori (sport judo) and horseback riding are among them.

Being a teacher, I will end this chapter with a story of one of my favorite martial arts students, my elder daughter (my younger went into gymnastics). After learning with me for several years, she quit, as students will. But in high school when she was physically attacked, she rising blocked to osoto gari and won a quick fight. It was her only high school fight.

My favorite Dojo memory of her was after class. She would pick up a bokken (wooden practice sword) and attack me. She would hit full out because she had confidence that she would not be able to hit me. As it happens she was correct. Just barely.

IN THE PRESENCE OF CHENG MAN-CH'ING

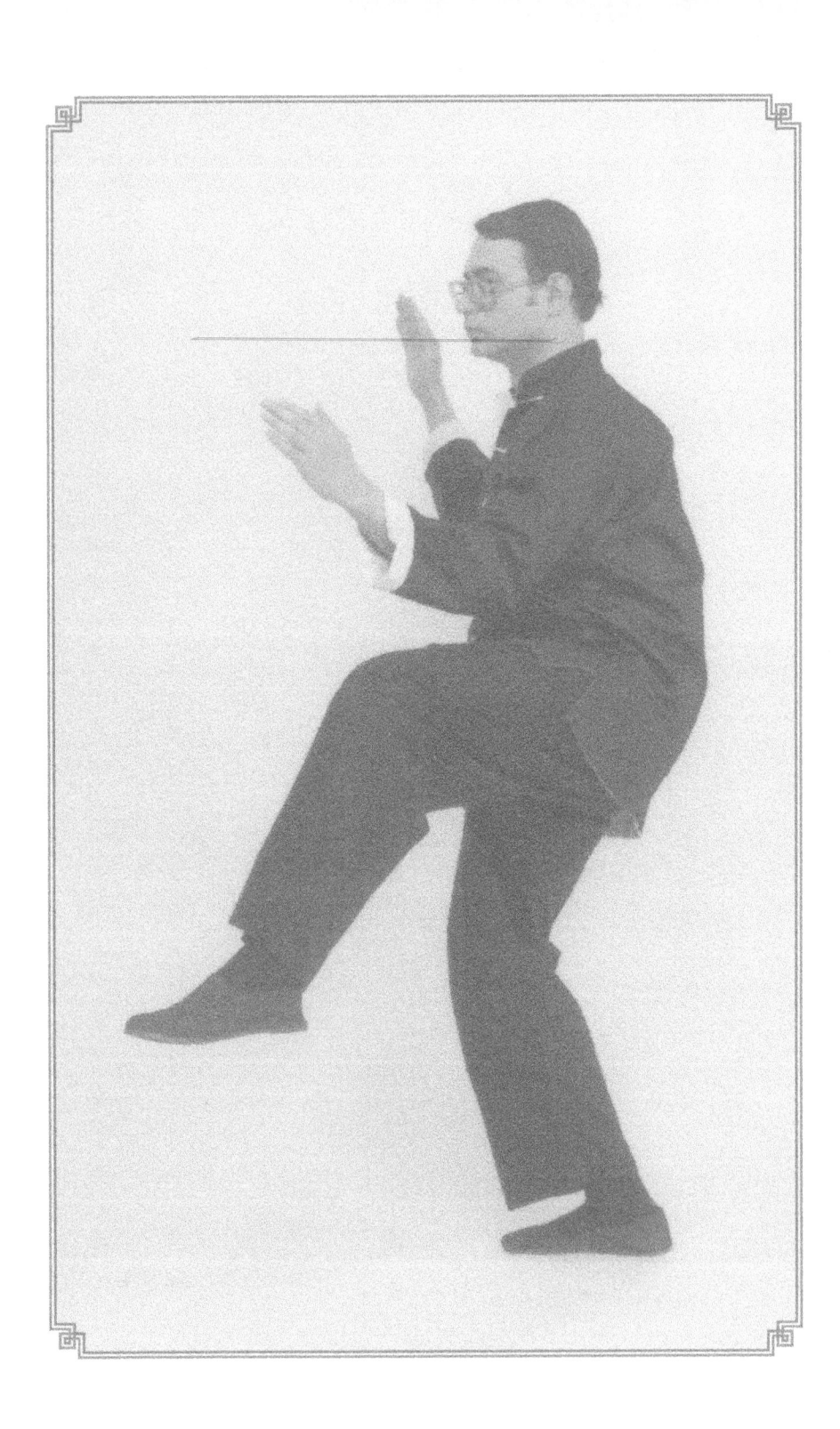

Chapter 14

Conclusion

IN THE END, TO SUM UP

It is funny that I started my T'ai Chi experience writing notes on scraps of paper, and now, about half way through my life, I again am resorting to notes on scraps of paper for this book. In some things we come full circle.

I have found so many notes and so much of Professor's wisdom as I unpacked while working on this book. If I have another book about Professor in me, should I have the time, I may produce a book just of the things in my notes and audiotapes.

ONE MAN CHANGED MY LIFE

It is often not easy to pick the one instant when your life is changed, and I am not sure in which instant it happened for me. I am sure of the man who caused it, though, and he is Professor Cheng Man–Ch'ing. He gave me T'ai Chi for the rest of my life, and I have benefited greatly. It has improved my movement skills and my balance and coordination, as well as my health. As a teacher, because of him, I have met many wonderful people, and have a T'ai Chi family both close, meaning my own students, and extended, meaning many wonderful classmates and colleagues.

Professor Cheng gave me ethics to live by, and an idea,

Chun-yun, to constantly measure my activities and relationships against. He gave me medicine for my health, and an appreciation of art, poetry, and calligraphy. He gave me ideas about philosophy, and the knowledge that you can think for yourself about what has been written.

He was also an example of a loving grandfatherly figure in my life. In my time at the T'ai Chi Association and the Shr Jung, the trajectory of my life changed, and changed for the better. What I am today is very much a result of that change.

When I began this journey I never thought I would write a book. I do not believe how much I have done so far in life, so if you don't either, well that makes two of us.

Often you study with someone and realize only after the fact they were a great teacher and that you were living though a really great time in your life. I was fortunate enough to know it when I lived it and that made things even more special.

FINAL THANK YOUS

Before going on to some classmates, I need to thank a very special person: That person is **Ohashi Sensei**, creator of Ohashiatsu, who worked on me monthly for five years, and biannually since. During the course of Elizabeth's and my treatments and Elizabeth's study of Ohashiasu, he befriended us. He is a wonderful living example of happiness, optimism and seeing through to the essence of things. He is also a gourmet chef.

And his wife **Bonnie Ohashi,** who is wonderful company and works hard to keep Ohashiatsu up and running so Ohashi Sensei can do the teaching and the treatments. I also wish to thank his son, **Kazu Ohashi**, who accompanies his father and is a combination of secretary, arrangement maker and appointment taker. There may be a lot more he does for his father that I do not know about.

At this point I ought to digress and thank **Dr. Sherek** and **Dr. Hume,** successive chairmen at Kingsborough Community College Department of Physical Education for making my time there seem like I was working in a heaven world.

And now some classmates:

Claire Hooten, who got me the job at Sheepshead Bay adult evening high school, which later moved over to Kingsborough Community College Division of Adult Education. As a result, I taught many years for them and finally for the College in a one credit course, PEC 25 T'ai Chi. I taught in the Physical Education Department from 1987 to 1995, and again from 2010 to 2015. Claire has also written a book on T'ai Chi.

Harold Naiderman, who did the electric wiring for the Shr Jung and helped me by installing electrical wiring and high-hat lights at Patience T'ai Chi on 10th Avenue in Brooklyn, our second location. (He let me help him as he worked, so I could learn something.) He was a good friend, and looked after the interests of the Cheng family

Jon Gaines, an advanced student who was a good friend and did carpentry. He worked on my house in Manhattan Beach Brooklyn, where I assisted him. In the process I learned some things about wood, and life. He then went on to have a center in Hawaii.

Lawrence Galante, a Shr Jung friend, who has a wonderful understanding of homeopathy. He has written a book on T'ai Chi, and, as of this writing, teaches T'ai Chi at Fashion Institute of Technology in New York City.

Lenny Antonucci, another Shr Jung friend, who rented me my first martial arts teaching location on 20th Avenue and 71st Street in Brooklyn. Later, when I was up for the teaching job at Kingsborough CC, he recommended me to them for it. Thanks, Lenny. And small world, he is also a friend of my friend Mario Napoli.

Kenneth Van Sickle. Without the "Official Photographer" of the Shr Jung and the Association, I would not have permission to print several of the photographs that are in this book. Thanks, Kenneth. He sells pictures of Professor Cheng, if you are interested. For those who wish to purchase one of his many pictures of Professor Cheng, he can be reached at http://sinobarr.com/ He, with Barry Strugatz, made the movie, The Professor, T'ai Chi's Journey West. It was an immense undertaking and I am grateful to them for interviewing me for the movie. I hope there will be a prequel and a sequel.

Robert Morningstar, who shared an advertisement in the Free Spirit Magazine with Marc Isaacs and myself. It was only $90 an issue, but that was a lot of money in those days, so sharing it made it work for the three of us.

I want to thank Mort Raphael's nephew, Steven, with who I played many pleasant hours of push hands.

To those whose names I may have forgotten, please forgive me, I ask that you contact me for a mention in future editions of this book if I get so lucky as to have them.

I want to thank some of those who are not with us any more, **Shep Shepard**, who was, for a time, my main push hands partner, and **Bataan and Jane Faigo** who moved to Colorado and taught Professor's T'ai Chi in the west. They did great things to advance Professor's T'ai Chi, and so thanks, fellow students.

I come now to thanking my colleagues, and T'ai Chi friends:

William C. C. Chen, his lovely wife Priscilla, and their children Max and Tiffany. William supported our Professor Cheng weekend and has always been there for me going back to the days when he would have guest speakers in his New York school. Patience T'ai Chi brought some benches and chairs to help accommodate the overflow of people. I always got a good seat, on the floor in front of the chairs or in the first row of seats. After one such class with Dr. Tao, I followed them to Atlantic City. He got me a room in a sold-out hotel, gave me coupons to eat for free, and asked me to take Dr. Tao to dinner, a wonderful honor. I still have my notes, written on a napkin, of our T'ai Chi discussion that night. As a result of William, I appear in a photo in Jonathan Russell's book about TT Liang's teachings, sitting and watching a TT Liang seminar at William's school.

A special word about Tiffany Chen, she has been a good acquaintance. I used to see her at tournaments, and have kept in touch on Facebook. She appeared doing T'ai Chi in the movie The Intern. Congratulations Tiffany.

I want to thank the late **Jou Tsung Hwa**, who was a wise man, an honorable man, and a good friend. He always shared whatever he was thinking, and he was almost always thinking about the principles of T'ai Chi. It was not until several years after he passed on that I realized just how profound some of his ideas were. For example: he had said that the form would teach me, and I had retorted that I had the teachings of Professor Cheng Man-Ch'ing and Zhang Lu-Ping, I could not learn T'ai Chi from the form. I was wrong. It is how I have improved in the 21st century: I am still making breakthroughs. I was just not ready then to hear Master Jou's wisdom, but fortunately I remembered. Master Jou created the Zhang San Feng event to bring all T'ai Chi and martial traditions together in a spirit of mutual harmony, respect, and learning. Something there is still not enough of today.

I thank the late **Sidney Austin**, who introduced me to Master Jou, and to **Angela Soucy** who has been a friend ever after.

I want especially to thank **Loretta Wollering**, who was a senior student of Master Jou's at the T'ai Chi Farm. She ran the day to day, and quietly made it a success for Master Jou. In Master Jou's tradition, she runs the T'ai Chi Gala in June, now in Pennsylvania. The Gala is the successor event to Master Jou's Zhang San Feng Festival and is dedicated to the memory of Master Jou. The event embodies the wish of Master Jou that all T'ai Chi and kung fu practitioners should live together and teach together, in harmony. For those who are interested in the event, which is a wonderful sharing space, you can contact me and I will give you Loretta's information. Oops, a brazen plug.

To **Dr. John Painter** who I met at many events, but mainly at the Zhang San Feng events and now at the Gala events, and who has been a friend these many years (well over 30 but since he looks so young, I better not say how many). Dr. Painter was always supportive of Master Jou and the Zhang San Feng event, and is now supportive of Loretta at the T'ai Chi Gala, as am I. If you show up at the Gala, take his class, you will not be sorry.

I want to thank **Mario Napoli**. As I was a student of Stan Israel's youth, he was a student of Stan's maturity. Stan brought him around to Patience T'ai Chi and we became friends. Mario won the Taiwan Championship, and took on all comers at the tournament and in the park the next day. He brought Professor Cheng's name back to mainland China by winning on the lei tai at Chen Village. Mario became a coach of my students and helped prepare them for many tournaments. He was also a speaker at our 100th Anniversary of the Birth of Professor Cheng. He is a good friend to all of us and very welcome at our Thursday night classes as well as the banquets we hold after class at Pacificana (now Pacific Palace) restaurant. He currently resides in Europe, but comes to the US to visit his

Mom and, when he does, stops by and visits us.

Another digression. Here I ought to thank **Jimmy, an owner of Pacific Palace,** who comes and sits with us, trades stories, and often personally takes our order. He sometimes sends a special dish over for our consideration. The restaurant is at 8th Ave and 55th Street in Brooklyn's Chinatown, over a Chase Manhattan Bank. The food is very good. That is another shameless plug in this book.

Diosdado Santiago, who pushed me to run the 100th Anniversary of the Birth of Professor Cheng Man-Ch'ing event. Without his asking me to do it and his constantly asking me how it was progressing, it may not have happened. Thank you, old friend. How old, you may wonder? We go back to the early T'ai Chi Farm days. He was also always available to teach T'ai Chi, massage and health, at my Holistic Weekends.

Friends from the T'ai Chi Gala:

Dale Dugas, who makes fantastic traditional dit da jou and who used to teaches at the T'ai Chi Gala. He is a very accomplished person in many things, and a very nice guy. His dit da jou is wonderful. Try it you will like it.

David Ritchie, another teacher and supporter of the T'ai Chi Gala, made the wonderful DVD, Riding with Chi with **Andrea Steele,** about the benefits of T'ai Chi in equestrian endeavors. It is the only DVD that I currently sell on the Patience T'ai Chi website that I did not make. He is my contact person in Connecticut.

I thank **Stephen Watson,** another wonderful T'ai Chi teacher and martial artist as well as a very wise and cheerful person. When we get together at events, the laughter just flows. Follow him on Facebook, and you too can partake of his wisdom.

Ken Lo, Wu Mai Pai lineage holder, and another practitioner who comes to the Gala. He also does an exquisite tea ceremony and tasting, and is a great guy.

Violet Lee, another Gala presenter who is a T'ai Chi journalist and shares fascinating articles on T'ai Chi with me.

Richard Clear, yet another teacher at the T'ai Chi Gala, though he is Tennessee based and it is a trip for him. He is a good practitioner and a gentleman of the Martial Arts.

And other friends throughout the T'ai Chi community:

Joanne Chang, who gets out a good newsletter about events all over the T'ai Chi community. When I met her, she was the wife of David Chen. Unfortunately this wise young man passed away. In his honor, Joanne, a gentle and loving soul, built the David Chen T'ai Chi Garden with private and public contributions in Cabin John Park, Montgomery County, MD, and she teaches there. Her T'ai Chi is excellent and she is my contact person in Maryland.

David Chen, Joanne's late husband who passed away far too soon, was always available to chat with about T'ai Chi. He was wise beyond his years. Joanne sells a book of some of his very perceptive sayings. Reach Joanne at Wuweitaichi.com.

Lee Scheele, who takes my west coast referrals and finds them teachers, and who came all the way across the country to the T'ai Chi Farm and my 100th Anniversary Celebration of the Birth of Professor Cheng Man–Ching.

Thanks to **Susannah DeRosa**, who made up the inventive T-shirt, "The Taoist Cowboys." After all these years, I still I wear it with joy in my heart. (It is the only T-shirt I wear, since I favor shirts with collars.) She supported Zhang Lu–Ping's events at Princeton.

Morgan Buchanan, author and T'ai Chi teacher and a student of Bill Law in Australia. He is a friend who warned me about the perils of self-editing this book, and always stops by when he is in the New York area. Morgan also gave me an out of print T'ai Chi book by one of Professor's students who I had done a seminar with at William C. C. Chen's place: J.J. Soong. Considering that we are both book collectors, it was an extraordinarily generous gesture. He has gone on to a career as a science fiction writer. He is currently collaborating with Claudia Christian. Wolfe's Empire is out. A second book is in the works, may it become a successful series. I wish him well. In addition, he is publishing this book.

I also want to thank:

Bill Law, Morgan Buchanan's teacher, who graciously helped me obtain T'ai Chi materials from mainland China.

Chris Luth, student of Abraham Liu, who teaches in Solana Beach, CA, and runs T'ai Chi in Paradise. He came to New York to teach at the 101st Anniversary of the Birth of Professor Cheng event.

The late **Robert W. Smith,** who was never so busy that he would not give me half an hour or so when I called to talk about his old days in Taiwan and gossip about the current state of T'ai Chi and the teachers that we knew.

And many more, including **Master Huang,** who runs the United States Kuo Shu Federation Tournament in Maryland, a wonderful event, and his student **John Green.** Also **Paul Ramos** who runs push hands rings at that event.

C.J. Rhoads in Pennsylvania, who is a founder and a driving force of the T'ai Chi Enthusiasts Organization. She also organizes the T'ai Chi Symposium, in New Jersey. She helps run the T'ai Chi Picnic in PA and works tirelessly for T'ai Chi.

Alan Goldberg, who runs the Action Martial Arts Hall of fame awards at the Tropicana Hotel and casino in Atlantic City, a wonderful event. We have been friends going back a long way.

Ged Moran in the United Kingdom, **Steve Levi** in Brooklyn, **Arnold Lenkersdorf** in Maryland, **Mike Daly** in Brooklyn, **Nathan Menaged** in Ohio, **Don Ethan Miller** in Connecticut, the late **Linda Schneiderman,** and **Wendy Cali,** north of New York City in Westchester, **Andy Lee** in New Jersey, **Don Schurman** in Idaho, **Toni Sardella** in upstate New York, **Tom Krapu** in St. Louis, **Gary Torres** in Florida, and **Andy Schirmacher** in New Jersey. I know that there are many more of you and I am sorry if I have left some of you out.

Then there are my own students: First, my very first student, **Peter Cerenzio.** Peter was a neighborhood, high school, and college friend. I invited him to study with me as a classmate, but he always said he would study with me when I started teaching. He kept his word. He came to class at our first location, on 20th Avenue, and then continued, and built the dressing rooms and the walls around the bathroom (for modesty of course) at the 10th Avenue place.

Thanks to the rest of the neighborhood High School gang, **Sal**

Martingano, Ernie Bono, Marty Siesta. Jerry Dinkels, and his cousin **Stewie Alexandrowitz.**

I wish to thank some of my other old students, going back to before I had "official" senior students, but these are some of the earliest senior students I ever had. **Marc Isaacs** on Long Island, who was loyal to me going back to our days in Shotokan Karate together, and came with me, when Avi Schneier could not, to visit Zhang Lu–Ping, towards the end of Master Zhang's life. **Richard Perpignand,** who ran the children's self-defense division of Patience T'ai Chi. He co-taught with me in the old days, and is now somewhere in Arizona. **Alex Marino,** currently in New Jersey, ex of Brooklyn, who taught at Paerdegat. When he was moving he gave the job to Marisa Coluccio, another of my students.

Then there are my more modern senior students:

Jim Leporati, acupuncturist, martial arts scholar, and TV personality with his own cable TV show, Martial Arts View. He began his study with me in 1981, and was my first official senior student. A tournament player in the 1980s, he became a coach of the Patience T'ai Chi (PTC) team in the 1990s and after. He is a wonderful senior student, and has always helped with teaching duties at PTC. It is not too much to say that PTC the school exists because Jim is reliably there on Thursday nights to teach and work with whoever may show up. In the days when I was unable to show up due to injury, he ran the school, and so the school was still there for me when I came back. Thank you Jim.

Avi Schneier, my second senior student, who has been a T'ai Chi form and push hands champion up and down the east coast as well as in England, and is, as of this writing, a chief judge at the USKSF (United States Kuo Shu Federation) tournament in Maryland. He does multiple styles of T'ai Chi as well as other martial arts. (He did ju jitsu under one of my black belt students, for example). For many years he also helped with the teaching at Patience T'ai Chi. I also thank his wife Natalia for putting up with Avi's being away so much on PTC's behalf. It is these two, Jim and Avi, who worked with me year in and year out, and were my right and left hands at Patience T'ai Chi in Brooklyn, cornerstones of my T'ai Chi family. Now that Avi is away for work and has moved to North Carolina,

Jim and I will have to make do without him. It is our loss.

Thanks to **Mike Pekor,** who has won 3 grand championships at the USKSF events in Hunt Valley MD, in addition to many other first place medals, and has his own school: T'ai Chi of Long Island (TaichilLi.com), and a hypnotherapy practice, also on Long Island. In his day job, he teaches Physical Education and T'ai Chi for the Physical Education Department of in a Long Island public school system. He is also a wing chun student of Sifu Crescione, an expert practitioner, a wonderful teacher, and a nice guy. Though busy with his own life and endeavors these days, Mike always stops by whenever he can to teach his push hands and wing chun skills to current students.

Jill Basso, now in Santa Fe, NM, teaches T'ai Chi and runs push hands workshops. She has won many medals in tournaments on the East Coast, and competed in Taiwan. She has appeared in magazines and newspapers (in several locales) as a proponent of T'ai Chi. She set up a school when she lived in the Hudson Valley in New York and left it to move and set up another school in Santa Fe. Recently, she was a presenter at the Symposium for the Integrative Health and T'ai Chi Retreat.

Marisa Coluccio, another medal winner, has taught in various places. In Brooklyn she taught at Paerdegat and she also taught in Far Rockaway. She also helps out at Patience T'ai Chi in Brooklyn. Marisa is always ready to assist wherever she is needed.

Zak Zaklad, who teaches in Philadelphia, PA is a very patient instructor. He is a therapist as well, teaching T'ai Chi to the disabled and helping them to recover. We met when he first came for a private class to brush up on CMC (Cheng Man–Ch'ing) form. He stayed when he saw the breadth of knowledge we could share with him. He also teaches karate and has written magazine articles thereon. He has a book of memoirs coming out. Zak runs seminars for Patience T'ai Chi in Philadelphia, and is our Philadelphia contact person.

Frime Kass, teacher—and assistant teacher when needed—as well as a Professor of Accounting at Brooklyn College. She does my taxes. Permit me a pun here, it is a very taxing job keeping up with my taxes. She helps me teach at Patience T'ai Chi as needed. She assisted me and taught at the

Chinese Scholars Garden in Staten Island back in the day.

Fred Mirer, retired high school history teacher, former teacher of T'ai Chi at the HEAP program at Brooklyn College and at the Staten Island Scholar's Garden. He is always ready to help with anything and assists with teaching at Patience T'ai Chi. I also thank his patient wife Charlotte, who does not complain when he is working or studying with us (or so we have heard).

The late **Cheryl Lindholm** who taught in Des Moines, IA. She stayed current and took private classes with me at every opportunity. She was a scholar who did many styles of T'ai Chi as well as other martial arts including judo. She often called and we shared our successes and aspirations over the telephone. She was also a retired nurse and an effective shiatsu therapist.

The late **Lyn Osloond**, retired teacher of T'ai Chi, who studied T'ai Chi with me via the internet and brought me out to Rapid City, SD, for final correction and to teach. She got me my first network TV interview on the ABC affiliate in Rapid City. She was a loyal friend. Thank you Lyn.

All family.

There are still more people to thank:

Kurt Griffith and his wife Heather, ex Brooklynites and former Nyack New York residents, now in West Virginia. Kurt was a student of my youth, at Midwood Judo Center. Then he came back to me in karate, judo, ju jitsu and T'ai Chi at Patience T'ai Chi years later. He did not know it then, but as my student at Patience T'ai Chi he taught me lessons about patience and loyalty which I still marvel at today. In addition, he did all the printing for the school and worked with me on the syllabus changes and the 20th anniversary party. He was always patient and loyal as teaching schedule changes were always messing with his life. He never complained when I, in similar circumstances, would have been screaming. Today he is earning dan rank in other systems and following the Native American spiritual path which is his heritage. I am very lucky that he and his wife are my friends, and were my students.

Rob Weber, a chiropractor and student of mine who pushed me to write this book. Yes, I was going to write it, but he kept asking me how it was coming until I had to answer him. So I got off my lazy a— and started writing. He also made a commitment to keep my back healthy and makes house calls when I need him. He is a wonderful friend. He asks wonderful questions.

Yes, Rob asks wonderful questions. This may give rise to the idea that Rob may sometimes not ask good questions, that would be wrong. Rob's questions are always good, the answers are sometimes deficient. Then, when I have had a chance to think about them, the answers do justice to the questions. The answers to some of those questions are paragraphs in this book.

In the same vein, **Mikhail Levitin**, student, friend, (brother by another mother), and his wife **Meri Stempel Levitin** his wife. Meri is my doctor and a friend, and Mikhail is a karate sensei, T'ai Chi sifu, inventor, multiple patent holder, physical therapist, and Olympic athlete (1980 Russian team). Mikhail rented space from me at Patience T'ai Chi to run his martial arts program and we became friends. When I did not have the price of a dinner after my child support and children's college payments were paid, Mikhail and Meri always invited me to their house and took me out to eat with them, and let me sleep there. It was my vacation home away from home. Mikhail Levitin teaches T'ai Chi in the Poconos, PA. In addition, for many years, and still, Mikhail fixed my back, patiently and with great expertise.

Sensei Thomas Casale, who, though certified to teach T'ai Chi, is much too successful with teaching karate and with being a high official in the Japan Shotokan Karate Association. He had an interview and cover in the April 2013 issue of Shotokan Karate Magazine. His dojo is in Brooklyn. Back in 1993, when I needed surgery to reattach my biceps tendon, he dropped his teaching duties in his own school to cover my classes when I could not be there. He is one of the few who, I find, understands the dynamics of striking techniques as I do them (or used to do them). I do not know if he learned them from me or another of his many stellar teachers, but he has them, and that is just wonderful.

John Leporati, Jim's brother, teaching wushu and T'ai Chi and high school English in Brooklyn. John helped me by setting up the original Patience T'ai Chi website. As a high school teacher at New Utrecht HS he dug up a copy of my student yearbook so we could look at my picture and laugh at how I had changed in the intervening years. He is a loyal and dedicated student and practitioner.

Carlos Martinez, the first student I met at Westinghouse V&T High School in 1970 in a class room on the first floor. He had a brown belt in karate, and though he was a student, he was my first Westinghouse martial arts buddy. He came to my school, I went to his. Finally, I sublet him space in the Sheepshead Bay School.

Donna Comanda, student and teacher of T'ai Chi on Staten Island, who got me and Patience T'ai Chi the job at the Chinese Scholar's Garden. In the small world department, she knows Guy Blackman and Mel Oliver, who were classmates of hers in nin jitsu under the late, world famous, Master Ronald Duncan.

Gregg Hammond in Peru, IN, **Tony Holmes** in Wabash, IN, teach T'ai Chi in Indiana. They are my Indiana guys, my Taiwan tournament team. Whenever I can get there they take me out and we have a good time.

Sal Casano, student of Marc Isaacs and myself, teaches T'ai Chi in Albany, NY. He shows up at the T'ai Chi Gala to enjoy, learn, and also to show support.

And I also thank a few more active students, who as of this writing, are not teachers.

Jim Black, a dedicated student at Patience T'ai Chi. He started with us in the Boro Park School and stayed with us. He provided the air conditioners and water cooler for the Sheepshead Bay School. While he left when we had to close down in Sheepshead Bay, he has returned to us at our newer location in Park Slope.

Larry Cummings and **Cathy Mulhy,** who come weekly and share our T'ai Chi and our banquets. Cathy helped with the editing of this book. She is a wonderful editor. And they are both good T'ai Chi friends and students.

Family all.

There are some students and teachers who rate mention mostly as friends.

Guy Blackman and **Mel Oliver**, amazing nin jitsu people, who started their martial arts with me. Mel started in the school on 20th Avenue, Guy in Borough Park. When Guy married Master Ronald Duncan's daughter, both Guy and Mel left to train in Guy's family system. They are both certified to teach T'ai Chi but so far have not. They are located in Queens and on Long Island. I have watched them grow from teenagers into men. They are loving family men, mature and caring individuals as well as powerful martial artists. They are two of my favorite people.

Alan Marks, who is Guy's cousin. He retired from the martial arts and is an attorney, and a mediator in Atlanta, GA.

Sue Terry, currently in Ecuador. Sue is a tournament champion, as well as a skilled saxophone player, and she plays many other instruments as well. She has written music instructional books, and published excerpts from her blogs as books: The Blog that Ate Brooklyn and For the Curious. When I asked her at the T'ai Chi Gala to just wing it and play something appropriate, I had no idea of just how hard that may have been, but she did it flawlessly.

Sam Sunshine, another musician, ex T'ai Chi student and a friend. He helped me move in 1988 (along with Kurt and Heather Griffith and Marcia Schackner). In 2014 he let us stay with him and his wonderful wife, Eileen when Elizabeth and I moved out of our apartment in Brooklyn until we got our mortgage and our new place ready.

Also, **Evie Graham** and her husband **Art McConnel**, on Long Island. **Miriam (Mimi) Delaglio** in Maryland, **Alan Klus** in Arizona, **Terry Wertan** in Georgia, **Lisa Rabinow Weber** in the Poconos, PA, **Roy Montalbano** in Mississippi, **Ira Resnick** in Texas, **Isiah Weiss, Sam Ida, Debbie Avodror,** and **Eli Dos Reiss**, in Brooklyn, **Cirilo Smith** of Vee Jitsu and the Judo and Karate Club of the United Nations, also in Brooklyn, **Joyce Finks** in Manhattan, and **Glen Mordecai and his wife, Debbie,** in Queens.

Craig Swanson who made dan rank with me, and then left, and, small world, now studies with Mike Pekor, on Long Island.

Nathan Belkowitz, Cathy Libraty, Frank Hechenberg, and Rick Ast, not sure where, and the late **Myron Slonim, his wife Harriet,** and many more of you throughout the years.

Artie Brown, an old friend who hunted for me, found me, and came back to renew our friendship after all these years. He is mentioned in this book.

Master Zhang Yuan, who graciously lets us have space in his T'ai Chi and Kung Fu school through two addresses.

Then these non–martial arts friends who influenced me to varying degrees:

First, at the Holistic Weekend I used to run:

Nicky and Ileana Velazquez, now mostly in Florida, without whom there could never have been much of a Holistic Weekend. Nicky did the desk and the printing, and Ileana patiently gave him to me, as well as helping at the desk. I met Nicky when he was a student at Westinghouse V&T High School, and I was his teacher. When I went on to become Cafeteria and Security Coordinator, he was on my service squad. Later, as we kept in touch, I watched him grow into a wonderful loving family man and a really good friend. They still have me over for barbecues and dinners when they are in Staten Island. I think I have become a part of the family.

Gus Carayas (and his late wife Peggy), my stretching and weight training teacher. I used to drive up to Middletown New York on Friday nights (when I was not needed at Patience T'ai Chi in Brooklyn), to exchange teaching T'ai Chi for learning Carayas Technique deep stretching and weight training. There I met and made a T'ai Chi instructor out of Toni Sardella as well, who was in Gus' classes. Gus has given me permission to get his stuff out and one day I will be selling his DVDs when I finally get around to it. (Or as we used to say at Westinghouse High School a round tuit, a very rare piece of wood indeed.)

Larry Heisler, my sometimes co-conspirator, speaker, and Holistic Weekend buddy. He was a student of Hilda Charlton, and a wonderful spiritual teacher he is, as well as a massage teacher, 5 laughter teacher, and so very much more. He runs the New Jersey School of Massage.

Joanne Ferdman was the Official Astrologer of the Holistic Weekend. She has also learned, and is a teacher of several other disciplines. She is a sweet woman who emails me her Astrology columns to this day.

Jan Krivoshiew–Wenz, the hypnotist and singles maven, who founded Singles for Charities. I joined the Board of Directors and helped out, but, in spite of Jan's help, could not find a date out of the whole organization. She helped me out by teaching hypnosis at the weekends.

Kathy Morley, a life-long friend who supported the event, and me. She got me an invite up to Su Casa to teach T'ai Chi, where I met Marilyn Raphael, among others.

Jeff Gold, who made and sold audiotapes for the weekend, and whose wife Carmel was a speaker. I see Jeff at various Expos where he is making CDs and DVDs of the speakers. He always has a good joke to tell you, just ask him.

Other friends, who taught me something:

Marilyn Raphael, wonderful friend and author of the book, Angelic Force. She has always has sound and timely advice for me when I ask for it, and sometimes even when I do not.

The late **Lyn Schroeder**, author of *Super Learning* and *Super Learning 2000*, who put me in the later book and spoke at our weekend. **Shabari Redbird Woman**, a very special speaker on Native American Culture and Spiritual practice, authors **Max Toth, Susun Weed**, (who often autographs her books on women's health to women, writing "Just in time" and autographed one to me "Just in case"). The late **Jean Munzer** of the New Jersey Metaphysical Center and her man, **Frank Ostrow**, who spread their wisdom at the events.

Janet Brennan, who runs psychic fairs and also gluten free events. She is also an expert seamstress and a very loyal friend.

Carla Tara, tantra teacher and author, who taught me the Ocean Breath and the Cobra Breath and many other ways to move energy that were not part of my traditional martial teachings. But they are very real and very useful, nevertheless.

Izzy Friedman, who taught me to have good look instead of trying to rely on good luck. He taught me a lot about how to be a good and spiritual person. Then we went to lunch at Garguilio's.

Tim Bracci, a more senior student of Izzy Friedman. Another dear friend, former ju jitsu student and speaker at the New Life Expo on crystals and stones.

Susan Kaufman, who is an adventurous and fun loving person. She is another special friend who shared her wisdom, and did her best to keep me balanced on my journey through life. The T'ai Chi never stuck, but so what.

Marcia Schackner is a life-long friend. In the early days at Patience T'ai Chi she assisted in the beginners' T'ai Chi. She also was a wonderful administrative assistant. She sat at the desk during many of the classes, taking money and keeping accurate records. In addition, in the children's classes, she comforted the children as needed and kept the parents informed. Along with Kurt and Sam she helped me move in 1988. Later she did all the artwork for my 60th birthday party, though unfortunately she was not able to attend.

Susan (Susy) Marmol, who threw my 50th and (with Elizabeth and Marcia) 60th birthday parties, thank you for always being there for me. I have known her for a long time, but from the look of her, you would never know it. She was a student too, but I won't say when she started for the same reason. You would not believe it to look at her anyway. Susy, I hope I get this book out before I turn 80. (I had 70 in mind, but that ship has sailed.)

Joyce Finks, T'ai Chi student at Kingsborough Community College. She went on to study ju jitsu, karate, and T'ai Chi at Patience T'ai Chi. She brings over a feast for the two of us every Thanksgiving.

The three aforementioned women, Marcia, Susy and Joyce, came to my aid when I was desperate. When my back went badly out, they all came to my house, each in turn, to bring food and prepare it. They helped me get up out of bed so I could function. They sat with me for the time they had so I was not so alone in those difficult days.

Josephine Bentley, her endlessly cheerful personality and optimistic outlook buoyed me through some difficult times.

Gail Thackray, a spiritual teacher and a friend, who is spreading spiritual healings and teachings throughout the world. It is my privilege to help her when she is in New York at the New Life Expo.

And then:

The late **Bea Aisenstark–Bonnes**, who had a healer's gift and an angel's heart. Who helped me learn to live with and begin to heal, both physically and emotionally, from a debilitating back injury received at work. In addition, she was a confidant and dear friend through a tough time in my life. This gentle soul showed me how to love, and for those of you who know me, if I hug well, thank her, it is because she taught me how.

And the late **Suzanne Himmel**, who was another special friend. When we met she was living in Long Beach, NY, then she moved to South Beach, FL. (A tale of two beaches?) We fought sometimes but she always forgave me. She was wonderfully enthusiastic about life. She taught me about being generous to one's children when they are in need. When she gave her son money she needed for her rent, she told me I could not understand because I was not a mother. I proudly escorted her to both of her children's weddings. She never quite learned the T'ai Chi I was trying to teach her, but I guess it really did not matter, after all.

And to close, family:

Jason Lubliner, my cousin and children's self-defense student, and his wife Susan.

Sometimes we save the best for the end. I take special note of and offer special thanks to **Elizabeth Crefin**, my dear, dear friend, lover, and life partner, who puts up with me (no small task). She is an assistant instructor at Patience T'ai Chi, helping with beginners and occasionally teaching T'ai Chi privately. Most weeks she drives me to and from the school. She fixes my computer and works on the web site. Without her gentle loving support, very little would get done, including this book.

My late Mom, who was always there for me, and my Dad, who passed away way too soon. And I mention **my sister Marcia, her kids David and Stacey**, and **my children Renee and Michelle, her husband Eric, and Renee's son Ryan, Michelle's sons Liam and Benjamin.**

And finally, **Bethanne "Wrenn" Simms**, my editor, who worked patiently with me as I went through this process. She is truly the midwife of this book, if it is actually born.

WILLIAM C. PHILLIPS

GLOSSARY

Bokken	A wooden sword used in Japanese martial arts.
Chin	Internal power. Jing in pinyin.
Kouchi gari	Judo throw where you sweep the foot in front of you forward from the inside.
Ch'i	Energy, also spelled chi. Qi in pinyin.
Chung-yung	The doctrine of the mean. Professor Cheng understood it as doing the exact appropriate amount at the exact right time.
Dan	Practitioner of a style who is usually recognized as a martial artist who has surpassed the kyū, or basic, ranks and become a black belt. They may also become a licensed instructor in their art.
Dojo	A martial arts school. Japanese, from dō 'way, pursuit' + jō 'a place'.
Fa chin	To issue or discharge power explosively. Fajin in pinyin.
Gi	Judo uniform.
Harai goshi	Hip throw with one foot in air, out side of the body of the uke (training partner).
Hane goshi	Hip throw with one foot in the air, lifting inside the leg of the uke.
Ippon Seoi Nage	Shoulder throw
Jing	A short sharp springy push

Judo	A Japanese martial art that primarily utilizes throws and locks.
Ju jitsu	A Japanese martial art practiced by samurai that is the predecessor of judo.
Karate	A Japanese Martial Art that primarily utilizes punches, blocks and kicks.
Kata	The pre-arranged pattern of movements in karate.
Kata guruma	Throw in which you pick your opponent up onto or over your shoulders and then let him fall from there.
Kuba nage	Tai otoshi except that your forearm is behind uke's head and as you trip him, you pull his head forward.
Kung fu	Chinese martial arts in general. A term that encompasses all styles. Also means a skill developed over time.
Lama	Tibetan Monk.
Llama	South American animal.
Matte	An instruction to wait or cease combat or practice in Japanese.
Nidan	Second black belt rank.
Nikkyu	Second grade of judo under black belt rank, brown belt.
Ninjitsu	Japanese martial art historically practiced by assassins.
O goshi	Hip throw.
Osoto gari	Major outer reap throw (sweep foot from outside).
Ouchi gari	Throw in which you sweep foot forward from inside.
Ouchi komi	Judo exercise, where you go in for the throw and then, with out throwing, withdraw from the throw. Therefore considered an "in and out" exercise.
Randori	Judo competition.
Sandan	Third black belt rank.
Savate	French martial art, known for kicking.

Sensei	Teacher (in this context, teacher of Japanese martial art).
Shinai	Japanese practice sword made of bamboo, it makes a loud noise but does not hurt to be hit with it.
Shodan	First black belt rank.
Shotokan	Style or method of karate.
Shr Jung	Name of the Professor's school.
Sifu	Teacher of Chinese Martial Arts.
Sumi gaeshi	Corner reversal throw in judo, a sacrifice technique.
T'ai Chi	Slow motion moving meditative exercise with health, and meditative benefits. It is also a martial art. Taiji in pinyin.
T'ai Chi Ch'uan	Full name of T'ai Chi, Ch'uan refers to boxing. Taijiquan in pinyin..
Tan t'ien	Point, approximately 1 inch under the navel, 1 ½ inside you. Dantien in pinyin.
Tai otoshi	Judo throw where you turn your back on your uke and put your right foot out and trip him.
Tomoe nage	Throw in which you sit in front of uke, stick a leg in their waist, sit and lift, throwing them over you (sacrifice technique)
Tai sabaki	Whole body movement or repositioning.
Torre	Person throwing the uke.
Uke	Person being thrown by torre.
Wing chun	A style of Chinese martial art.
Yonkyu	Fourth rank under black belt, green belt.

WILLIAM C. PHILLIPS

TERMINOLOGY

Senior student — Student who is senior to most others and also takes some responsibility for helping the teacher and the school.

To slap out — To give up, surrender.

Green belt — Rank after yellow in the system I was in.

Yellow belt — Rank after white belt.

White belt — Beginner's rank, when you first start.

APPENDIX 1

School principal's letter of thanks after the author disarmed an agitated, knife-weilding student.

BOARD OF EDUCATION OF THE CITY OF NEW YORK

George Westinghouse VOCATIONAL AND TECHNICAL High School

105 JOHNSON STREET, BROOKLYN, NEW YORK 11201   MAIN 5-6130

April 14, 1975

Norman Shapiro
Principal

Mr. William Phillips
Cafeteria Coordinator

Dear Mr. Phillips:

    I want to commend you and make a matter of record your subduing and disarming a disturbed knife-wielding student in the students' cafeteria last Thursday.

    You demonstrated leadership, personal courage, and appropriate behavior which is not covered by any set of written standard operating procedures. You were truly a teacher-in-charge, a fact noted by all the students who saw you take actions in a highly charged situation.

    I want you to know that I appreciate the stress and tension of the total situation you faced. On behalf of the entire school community, I want to thank you.

Sincerely

Norman Shapiro
Principal

NS:em
cc: Teacher's File
    Mrs. Roxee W. Joly, Assistant Superintendent

AUTHOR'S BIOGRAPHY

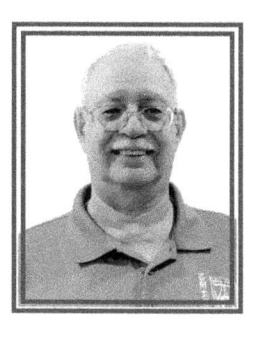

William C. (Bill) Phillips began his study of martial arts in 1965, when it looked like his college classmates were having so much fun hip throwing each other into the couch that he wanted to join them. Several years later, his judo and jiu–jitsu teacher, Stanley Israel, spoke of a larger–than–life, little old man in New York City's Chinatown who could perform incredible martial feats, but Stanley refused to reveal his location. Bill eventually had to seek out this man and went knocking on doors in Chinatown until he found Professor Cheng Man–Ch'ing, and also found that all the amazing stories, and then some, were true.

Bill's studies with Professor Cheng and the teaching of his own students were nearly thwarted in the early 1970s when his father pressured him to give up his school and studies to follow his footsteps into law. When Bill proposed instead to give up his job as a high school English teacher and continue his martial arts career while going to law school, his Dad simply replied, "You're not hungry enough." Today, the hundreds of students Bill has taught t'ai chi, karate, and ju jitsu to since he opened Patience T'ai Chi in 1970 thank him for making the right decision and openly sharing his knowledge and love of these arts for all these years.

Bill currently resides in the Bronx with over 4,000 books, file cabinets filled with articles he and his students have published, VHS tapes and the DVDs of thousands of movies and a respectable number of recordings of his own appearances on TV shows around the USA, countless plaques and awards, and his loving wife, Elizabeth, who wonders where to put it all. For more information or to arrange a workshop, seminar, or private lesson, please go to PatienceTaiChi.com or contact the association directly below:

William C. Phillips, Patience T'ai Chi Association
PO Box 630001, Bronx NY 10463
Email: sifu@patiencetaichi.com

Lightning Source UK Ltd.
Milton Keynes UK
UKHW010603100320
360054UK00002B/60/J